HEALTH CARE POLICY IN THE UNITED STATES

edited by

JOHN G. BRUHN
PENNSYLVANIA STATE
UNIVERSITY-HARRISBURG

A GARLAND SERIES

Health Care Policy in the United States
John G. Bruhn, editor

CAN EFFICIENCY AND COMMUNITY SERVICE BE SYMBIOTIC?

A Longitudinal Analysis of not-for-profit and for-profit Hospitals in the United States

SHARYN J. POTTER

GARLAND PUBLISHING, INC.
A MEMBER OF THE TAYLOR & FRANCIS GROUP
NEW YORK & LONDON/2000

Published in 2000 by
Garland Publishing, Inc.
A member of the Taylor & Francis Group
29 West 35th Street
New York, NY 10001

Copyright © 2000 by Sharyn J. Potter

10 9 8 7 6 5 4 3 2 1

Library of Congress Cataloging-in-Publication Data
Potter, Sharyn J.
    Can efficiency and community service be symbiotic? : a longitudinal analysis of not-for-profit- and for-profit hospitals in the United States / Sharyn J. Potter
        p. cm— (Health care policy in the United States)
    Includes bibliographical references and index.
    ISBN 0-8153-3633-0
    1. Hopital and community—United States—Longitudinal studies. 2. Voluntary hospitals—United States—Longitudinal studies. 3. Hospitals, Proprietary—United States— Longitudinal studies. I. Title. II. Series.

RA965.5 .P67 2000
362.1'1'0973

                                99-055076

Printed on acid-free, 250 year-life paper
Manufactured in the United States of America

For Mike, Audrey and Shelly

Contents

List of Tables and Figures

Acknowledgements

This book has benefited from the intellectual and emotional support of many wonderful professors, friends and family. However, I take full responsibility for any remaining deficiencies.

I would like to thank faculty from the Emory University Department of Sociology and the Rollins School of Public Health of Emory University. Karen Hegtvedt and Alex Hicks provided direction, support and suggestions on earlier versions of the manuscript. Tim Dowd continuously challenged me to think about my question in a theoretical framework. As a supportive mentor Dick Levinson attended my ASA presentations at ungodly hours in the morning. I hope that in the future I can emulate his qualities as a caring teacher.

I would especially like to thank my mentor Edmund (Ned) R. Becker for his insight, patience, friendship and sense of humor. I have enjoyed working with Ned for the past six years. During this period I have learned a great deal about research, teaching and politics. I will never forget these lessons, and I will always look back at these times with fondness and appreciation.

I would also like to thank E. Kathleen Adams for being both a mentor and a wonderful friend. The quality and depth of my work evolved through discussions that took place while running and over meals of gummy bears and burritos. I am also grateful to Patrick Mauldin for his encouragement and for his advice to treat graduate school like a full time job in corporate America.

My book has also had the benefit of special friends including Laurel Pickering who introduced me to the Rollins School of Public Health of Emory University and who has encouraged my research endeavors in the health care field. Sunday brunches with Amy Conti Harkness and her son Erik started during our Masters in Public Health program and continued for the next four years brightened many Sundays that were spent in the library. Kris Principe constantly provided me with the benefit of her experience as a doctoral student and was always there to listen and give both advice and friendship. I also thank Margie Pintzow for her support and her many gifts of chocolate during periods of celebration and frustration. Finally, I thank my best friend for the past seventeen years, Liz Krauss for her support. Liz even moved to Atlanta to pursue a Masters in Physical Therapy so we could spend two years in the same city as we pursued our educational goals. I hope I am able to give back to all of you what you have given me in terms of your support and friendship.

I would also like to thank the members of my family who were always a phone call away and moved around family vacations and celebrations to accommodate my work schedule. In particular, I would like to thank my brother Jeremy Potter and my sister Elyse Levy for their love, support and constant encouragement. My parents Audrey and Shelly Potter deserve more thanks than I can ever possibly express. They have constantly told me that I can do anything that I set my mind on. With these directions they have always been there with love and encouragement and an ear to listen.

Finally, I would like to thank Mike Schwartz for his love, support and patience. Mike has been there since the beginning of this endeavor and has made this journey a special one. Mike has constantly encouraged me to follow my dreams and has been supportive, as these dreams have sometimes led us down unexpected paths. I hope that in the future I can give Mike the same freedom to follow his own dreams.

I realize that these acknowledgements only touch the surface of my deep appreciation and gratitude to all of you for so many different reasons. I know that my career and my personal life has, and will always be enriched from my experiences with all of you. Thank you again.

Sharyn J. Potter

CAN EFFICIENCY AND COMMUNITY SERVICE BE SYMBIOTIC?

A LONGITUDINAL ANALYSIS OF NOT-FOR PROFIT AND FOR-PROFIT HOSPITALS IN THE UNITED STATES

CHAPTER 1
Introduction

In his 1982 Pulitzer Prize-winning book chronicling American medical history, *The Social Transformation of American Medicine*, Paul Starr cautions that consolidation in the medical industry will make voluntary not-for-profit hospitals indistinguishable from their for-profit counterparts:

> The extension of the voluntary hospital into the profit-making businesses and the penetration of other corporations into the hospital signal the breakdown of the traditional boundaries of voluntarism. Increasingly, the polycorporate hospitals are likely to become multihospital systems and competitors with profit-making chains, HMOs, and other health care corporations . . . Eventually, it may also be difficult to distinguish those health care conglomerates that began as hospital systems from those that began in other markets[1]

In recent years, numerous researchers echo Starr's assertion that the once-salient distinctions between not-for-profit and for-profit hospitals are quickly eroding.[2] Researchers find minimal differences between for-profit and not-for-profit hospital outcomes when comparing the types of patients served, the ratio of medical staff to hospital beds, the availability of onsite training for hospital personnel, operating costs and hospital size.[3] These converging outcomes represent a striking departure from past differences. Historically, not-for-profit hospitals were larger and treated a higher proportion of seriously ill patients than for-profit hospitals. Not-for-profit

hospitals also had larger medical staffs and offered greater opportunities for medical training. These characteristics of not-for-profit
hospitals, in turn, made for higher operating costs than at for-
profit hospitals.[4]

Researchers have vigorously debated the implications of the
fading distinction between for-profit and not-for-profit hospitals.
As these researchers note, numerous communities support not-
for-profit hospitals with taxpayer dollars, income and property-tax
exclusions and tax-free financing and contributions. Many are
concerned that not-for-profit hospitals will jettison community
service in an attempt to reduce operating costs.[5] Despite such
important implications this literature is full of philosophical discussions, typically employing limited empirical data, of the plight
of the not-for-profit hospital in the costly medical arena.[6] Furthermore, most of the empirical research examines cross-sectional data
or data representing a limited time frame.[7] In other words, the
researchers are trying to develop a historical argument, but their
assessments lack longitudinal data that allow for trend analyses.

To be sure, a group of researchers empirically demonstrate
that not-for-profit hospitals and for-profit hospitals are converging in a number of ways.[8] Most of these researchers, however, ignore
environmental pressures that may promote such convergence.[9]
Typically, they examine the hospital's internal structure while over-
looking its environment. The few researchers who actually consider the environment typically examine only one facet. Hultman,
for example, documents that the implementation of the 1983 Prospective Payment System prompted not-for-profit and for-profit
hospitals to offer similar amounts of charity care.[10] Norton and
Staiger find that for-profit hospitals seek to locate in more affluent
areas to ensure a lower demand for charitable care.[11] This limited
consideration of environmental factors (i.e., policy, supply and
demand) leaves an important question unanswered: How do environmental factors *combine* to produce the narrowing distinction
between not-for-profit and for-profit hospitals?

The research examines the claims of a narrowing distinction
between not-for-profit and for-profit hospitals by analyzing hospital outcomes over a fifteen-year period. Prior researchers have not
used this long a time frame, and, hence, their studies may not capture the development of certain trends. They have also limited their
analysis to a few states; this research uses data from every short-

term general hospital in the 48 contiguous states. Therefore, the results will capture national trends rather than just regional trends.

This book proceeds in six chapters. Chapter 2 reviews organizational theories that posit significant environmental influence on organizations. Drawing on neo-institutional theory, the effects of environmental and internal factors on hospital efficiency and community service outcomes are examined. A historical and analytical overview of the not-for-profit/for-profit distinction in the hospital industry is also provided. Chapter 3 provides the analytical layout of this research project, describing the data and the dependent variables. The dependent variables include two indices of hospital efficiency and two indices of community service. Chapter 4 provides an overview of the internal and external factors controlled for in this research. The internal factors include hospital affiliation, hospital size, teaching status and case mix; the environmental factors are physician mix, location, population demographics and indices of community wealth. Chapter 5 provides an in-depth description of the procedures used to merge internal and environmental characteristics and an explanation of the research methods. The results of the study are presented in Chapter 6. Additionally, the final chapter addresses the broader implications of this research and explains how these findings relate to current healthcare policy.

NOTES

1. Paul Starr, *The Social Transformation of American Medicine* (New York: Basic Books, 1982), 438.

2. See Rosemary Stevens, *In Sickness and In Wealth: American Hospitals in the Twentieth Century* (New York: Basic Books, 1989); M. L. Fennel, and J. A. Alexander, "Perspectives on Organizational Change in the US Medical Sector, 7 *Annual Review of Sociology* 19 (1993): 89–112.

3. R. E. Herzlinger, and W. S. Krasker, "Who Profits from Nonprofits?" *Harvard Business Review* (1987) 93–105; B. Arrington, and C. C. Haddock, "Who Really Profits from Not-For-Profits?" *Health Services Research* 25 (1990): 291–304.

4. Starr, *The Social Transformation of American Medicine;* Stevens, *In Sickness and In Wealth;* Lawton R Burns, "The Transformation of the American Hospital: From Community Institution toward Business Enterprise," *Comparative Social Research* 12 (1990): 77–112.

5. Nancy Kane, "Report on the Financial Resources of Major Hospitals in Boston." (Department of Health and Hospitals, Boston 1993); M. A. Morrisey, G. J. Wedig and M. Hassan, "Do Nonprofit Hospital Pay Their Way?" *Health Affairs* 15 (1996): 132–144.

6. See H. P. Tuckman and C. Y. Chang, "A Proposal to Redistribute the Cost of Hospital Charity Care," *The Milbank Quarterly* 69 (1991): 113–141; Fennel and Alexander, "Perspectives on Organizational Change in the US Medical Sector."

7. C. Y. Chang and H. P. Tuckman. "The Profits of Not-For-Profit Hospitals," *Journal of Health Politics, Policy and Law* 13 (1988) 547–64; Nancy Kane, "Report on the Financial Resources of Major Hospitals in Boston."

8. Herzlinger and Krasker, "Who Profits from Nonprofits;" Chang and Tuckman, "The Profits of Not-For-Profit Hospitals."

9. Herzlinger and Krasker, "Who Profits from Nonprofits;" Chang and Tuckman, "The Profits of Not-For-Profit Hospitals;" Arrington and Haddock, "Who Really Profits from Not-For-Profits?"

10. Cheryl I. Hultman, "Uncompensated Care before and after Prospective Payment: The Role of Hospital Location and Ownership," *Health Services Research* 26 (1991): 614–22.

11. E. C. Norton, and D. O. Staiger, "How Hospitals Ownership Affects Access to Care for the Uninsured," *Rand Journal of Economics* 25 (1994): 171–85.

CHAPTER 2

Organizational Theory and the Orientation of Not-For-Profit and For-Profit Hospitals

ORGANIZATIONAL THEORY AND THE ENVIRONMENT

This research relies on neo-institutional theory. Neo-institutionalists study how environmental factors promote a declining distinction between organizational types. These theorists find that different types of organizations adopt similar strategies to meet the demands of their changing environments.[1] Before describing the theory in detail, a brief illustration is provided to show how neo-institutional theory builds on and extends previous organizational research.

Historical Overview of Organizational Theory and the Environment

The prevailing concern with environmental factors in organizational behavior reflects longstanding trends in organizational theory. In fact, the evolution of organizational research testifies to the importance of various environmental factors. Since the 1950s and 1960s, organizational researchers have grappled with various environmental factors when explaining organizational outcomes. Consider the following brief description of the environmental factors stressed in the organizational literature.

The strategies that personnel in organizations use to adjust to environmental changes have intrigued organizational theorists since the publication of Philip Selznick's seminal work on the Tennessee Valley Authority (TVA).[2] Arguing that organizations must deal with sources of power beyond their boundaries, Selznick demonstrated that TVA personnel had to compromise their original goals to satisfy the concerns of these interest groups. By altering their original goals, TVA personnel were able to maintain the viability of their organization. A stream of research in this tradition includes Zald and Denton's study of the Young Men's Christian Association's (YMCA) and Messinger's study of the Townsend organization. Like Selznick, Zald and Denton and Messinger illustrate how organizations, the YMCA and the Townsend organization, respectively, survived environmental changes and found new missions to ensure the organizations' future.[3]

In the mid- to late 1960s, contingency theorists continued Selznick's focus on the environment. These theorists, however, were not interested in the influence of interest groups; instead they studied how environmental uncertainty influences organizational structure.[4] When structuring an organization, they asserted, managers should focus on environmental uncertainty. Organizations that perform routine tasks, for example, should be highly bureaucratic. Alternatively, organizations that perform more nonroutine tasks should be decentralized, with little hierarchy.[5] Researchers have found that decentralization facilitates creativity and ingenuity in organizations specializing in complex technology (e.g. NASA).[6]

In the 1970s, resource dependency theorists also focused on environmental uncertainty, examining how organizations take action to minimize such uncertainty. Unlike contingency theorists, resource dependency theorists argued that organizations are decisively affected by the behaviors of other organizations—including competitors, customers, and suppliers—that have the potential to create environmental uncertainty. For instance, the introduction of revolutionary products forces existing organizations to revise their product strategies (e.g., the introduction of Microsoft Windows). Resource dependency theorists found that organizations often attempt to reduce environmental uncertainty by means of interorganizational linkage mechanisms which range from networks to joint ventures.[7] Through such linkages, for example, separate organizations can collaborate on the creation of new products. Resource dependency theorists—like Selznick and contingency theorists - portray organizations as adapting to challenges posed by the environment.

Contingency perspectives and resource dependency perspectives presently dominate hospital research. However, Alexander and colleagues assert that both approaches probably overestimate the ability of management to control the external environment.[8] They use the example of surgical treatment for kidney stones to explain their position: "As methods for treating kidney stones become more diverse, successful exploitation of this cluster [of kidney stone treatment services] becomes more difficult. Other institutions may offer a less painful, more expeditious method of curing kidney stones such as laser treatments."[9] Therefore, once-successful strategies such as price variation and hospital amenities may become ineffective in the face of recent environmental changes.

Population ecology emerged in the late 1970s to offer a new perspective on how environments influence organizational outcomes. Employing an evolutionary approach, population ecologists posit that the environment eliminates those organizations that do not fit.[10] An organization's survival is dependent on its standing in relation to its competitors and to the environmental forces that influence that population. Consequently, population ecologists conceptualize the environment as consisting of resources. They argue that these resources enable organizations to perpetuate themselves, and that the organizations that are best adapted to securing resources will survive.[11] Those organizations that are unable to secure resources will cease to exist or will only survive in changed forms.[12] As Alexander and his colleagues suggest, this theory offers a corrective to past approaches: it emphasizes the powerful impact of the environment to which organizations may not always successfully adapt.

Neo-institutional theory—a relatively new perspective in the organizational literature—also relies on environmental factors to explain organizational outcomes, building on and extending the theories described above.

Overview of Neo-Institutional Theory

Neo-institutional theory stresses both the powerful impact of the environment like previous theories, but it also notes the adaptive capability of organizations. Consequently, this theory and its resulting research provide a foundation for the present study. Like Selznick, neo-institutional theorists study how external factors affect organizational outcomes.[13] Neo-institutionalists, however, focus not on local interest groups but on the larger environment.[14] Among other things, they analyze how federal and state regulations affect organizational outcomes. Like contingency theory, neo-institutional theory investigates why organizations alter their behaviors in different environmental climates. Unlike contingency theory, neo-institutional theory does not overestimate the ability of management to control its environment through organizational structuring. Neo-institutionalists argue that organizational personnel tend to borrow familiar structures from other industries regardless of their applicability to the organizational task. Therefore, attempts to adopt new organizational structures are sometimes inefficient or less than optimal. Similar to resource dependency theorists and population ecologists, neo-institutional theorists consider the influence of competitors, suppliers and customers. However, neo-institutional theory broadens its scope to encompass relevant organizations outside the organization's network and organizations in other industries, including suppliers, competitors, distributors and federal, state and local governments.[15] Furthermore, neo-institutionalists study how environmental factors promote narrowing distinctions between organizational types. Neo-institutionalists identify three mechanisms that spur organizational similarities: coercive isomorphism, mimetic isomorphism and normative isomorphism.[16] Their focus on organizational convergence obviously resonates with the current debate on hospitals described in the previous chapter.

Coercive Isomorphism

According to DiMaggio and Powell, coercive isomorphism "stems from political influence and the problems of legitimacy."[17] Simply put, regulatory changes often force differing organizations to pursue similar strategies, which tend in turn to lead to similar organizational outcomes.[18] DiMaggio and Powell explain that legitimacy represents an organization's desire to ensure that it can provide the same benefits and services as its competitors. For instance, many small accounting firms offer a broad range of services that are not cost-effective. These services may require expensive equipment and personnel. However, the owners of small firms feel that, by offering the same services as larger firms, they have legitimately established themselves as viable competitors. Furthermore, Estes and Swan demonstrate that organizational affiliations, like regulatory changes, force different organizational types to pursue similar strategies, leading to similarities in organizational outcomes by comparing independent home health agencies with home health agencies that are affiliated with for-profit and not-for-profit systems.[19]

The diffusion of personnel departments represents an example of coercive isomorphism.[20] Widespread adoption of these departments occurred during World War II because the federal government wanted to reduce the labor shortages and turnovers caused by wartime production. As a result, new legislation mandated that employees have official certificates to change jobs. Firms responded by creating personnel departments to monitor employee certification and turnover. These departments were widely adopted across all industries during World War II as a result of environmental factors rather than internal factors. Other research dramatically shows that regulatory changes coerce convergence in organizational outcomes.[21]

In the hospital industry, the 1983 implementation of the Prospective Payment System (PPS) is an example of coercive isomorphism. This legislation enabled the federal government to determine hospital prices for Medicare. Prior to the passage of PPS, individual hospitals set prices. Following the implementation of the PPS, some researchers found that different types of hospitals adopted similar strategies. For instance, Hultman found that not-for-profit and for-profit hospitals in the same geographic areas provided different amounts of charitable care before the implementation of this legislation but similar amounts thereafter.[22]

Mimetic Isomorphism

DiMaggio and Powell refer to imitative responses to uncertainty as mimetic isomorphism: "When goals are ambiguous, or when the environment creates symbolic uncertainty, organizations may model themselves on other organizations."[23] To minimize risk during times of uncertainty, organizations imitate the strategies of successful organizations in their environment.

The college-textbook publishing industry illustrates the mechanism of mimetic isomorphism. Experienced editors in the industry indicate that there are no identifiable steps certain to lead to success. As a result, editors tend to imitate features of previously successful textbooks.[24] Other research demonstrates that organizations often imitate other organizations that are pursuing successful strategies.[25]

Mimetic isomorphism is widespread in the hospital industry. In recent years, for-profit hospitals have experienced extraordinary growth in their earnings. For-profit hospital stocks have outperformed other industry stocks (e.g. retail, aerospace) in the past decade. The growth of Hospital Corporation of America (HCA), a for-profit hospital chain, is one example of this phenomenon. The stock price of HCA has risen at more than twice the rate of Standard and Poor's 500 in the past six years.[26] Traditionally, not-for-profit hospitals have been less profitable than for-profit hospitals. Not-for-profit hospitals have also had higher medical-personnel-to-hospital-bed ratios than their for-profit counterparts. Recent data on acute-care hospitals, mostly from Florida, "suggest that the pattern of higher profits and reduced staffing at for-profit hospitals has persisted."[27] In recent studies, the staffing ratio has been used as a measure of hospital efficiency.[28] In an attempt to maximize profits, not-for-profit hospitals are mimicking the efficiency strategies of their for-profit counterparts by reducing the ratio of medical personnel per hospital bed. This is an example of how not-for-profit hospitals imitate the successful strategies of their for-profit counterparts.

Normative Isomorphism

Normative isomorphism is organizational convergence generated by professionals and professional associations.[29] DiMaggio and Powell "interpret professionalization as the collective struggle of members of an occupation to define the conditions and methods of their work."[30] The diffusion of strategies through professional associations, journals and turnover contributes to similarities in organizational outcomes. Research illustrates the profound effects of normative isomorphism.

U.S. art museums offer one example of normative isomorphism.[31] Funding sources were scarce for the education of museum personnel prior to the 1920s. Lack of resources prohibited museum personnel from establishing a strong professional association; the activities of their association, the American Association of Museums, were limited to lectures on museum philosophy.[32] Then a grant from the Carnegie Corporation in 1929 funded specialized training programs for museum personnel. As personnel from a wide variety of museums received training at the same programs, museum operations across the country became standardized.

Similarly, the development of the Joint Commission on the Accreditation of Healthcare Organizations (JCAHO) has promoted normative isomorphism in the hospital industry. Since 1952, the JCAHO, a not-for-profit organization, has been developing hospital accreditation standards.[33] Loss of accreditation from the JCAHO can be detrimental to hospital operations. For instance, hospitals must meet JCAHO accreditation standards in order to participate in the Medicare program, an important source of income.[34] Whatever their profit orientation, hospitals have thus adopted standardized practices in order to meet JCAHO standards.

Applying Neo-Institutional Theory

The mechanisms of institutional isomorphism provide insight into similar organizational outcomes. Neo-institutional theory suggests that organizations in comparable environments will have similar outcomes.[35] Therefore, the declining distinction in the hospital industry may be largely a function of new regulatory developments and increased market pressures that spur imitation. In order to apply the predictive power of neo-institutional theory, we need to study these phenomena.

This research investigates whether the hospital industry is consistent with the findings of past neo-institutional research. In particular, the author argues that the changing regulatory environment has forced different types of hospitals to adopt similar strategies that result in similar outcomes. Before describing the specifics of the hypotheses, the analytical and historical differences among four types of hospitals are discussed.

ORIENTATIONS OF FOR-PROFIT
AND NOT-FOR-PROFIT HOSPITALS

The Analytical Distinction Between For-Profit and Not-For-Profit Hospitals

The major distinction between for-profit and not-for-profit hospitals involves the distribution of profits. For-profit hospitals can distribute profits to their owners or shareholders. Therefore, stock-holders demand that for-profit hospitals should behave in a man-ner that results in healthy financial statements.[36] Furthermore, Homer and colleagues explain that these well-defined profit goals are the most appropriate justification for policies that tend to exclude poor patients. Indeed, Bradford Gray argues that prof-itability is the key indicator for evaluating the success of a for-profit hospital: "The penalties that managers pay for disappointing earn-ings range from a decline in the value of their own stock, to the loss of their jobs, to the possibility that the company itself will cease to exist as an independent entity."[37]

Not-for-profit hospitals can also earn profits, but they are pro-hibited from distributing these profits. Instead, profits must be re-invested in the hospital. Therefore, these hospitals "have historically had an aura of community service rather than profit seeking."[38]

Most hospital research neglected to look at profit orientation until 1976, when William Rushing argued that an organization's profit orientation influences organizational outcomes.[39] Rushing asserted that for-profit hospitals focus on market and economic criteria, and that not-for-profit hospital's criteria are more ambigu-ous. Not-for-profit hospitals, for instance, focus on how well they are meeting the health-care needs of their communities. According to Rushing, for-profit organizations find it easier to make formal assessments, because they use concise economic criteria. It is easy, for example, to determine the amount by which a hospital's in-come exceeds its operating expenses. It is far more difficult to measure the hospital's impact on the health of a target popula-tion.[40] Researchers have demonstrated the salience of the orienta-tion toward profit in other industries.[41] Consistent with Rushing's assertions, this study will analyze organizational outcomes in light of internal factors, including the hospital's profit orientation, and external factors in the hospital's environment to determine whether these factors are influential in determining hospital efficiency, and the hospital's provision of community care.

The Historical Distinction Between For-Profit and Not-For-Profit Hospitals

Let us examine how the analytical distinction between for-profit and not-for-profit hospitals have played out historically, by examining their origins, their present situation and the controversies facing these two types of institutions.

The Not-For-Profit Hospital Sector

The not-for-profit hospital sector can be further subdivided into the private not-for-profit sector and the government not-for-profit sector. Throughout American medical history, these two sectors have met different needs.

The private not-for-profit hospital sector. Private not-for-profit hospitals are operated by private and religious organizations. Religious hospitals were "organized and supported both out of fear and mistrust of the larger society, and because of special services they offered their own people. Like churches and fraternal organizations, hospitals were agencies of identification for uprooted immigrants, promoting group cohesiveness."[42] Not-for-profit government hospitals, are considered a separate category because of their different funding structures as the bulk of the funding for these hospitals is tax based, and they are subject to different financial pressures than their private not-for-profit counterparts.[43]

As early as the 1900s, not-for-profit hospitals combined business and voluntarism, not withstanding what Stevens calls the "current myth" that American not-for-profit hospitals historically provided their services for free[44]. Since 1913, the federal government has exempted not-for-profit organizations from most revenue and property taxes. In exchange for their tax exemption, these hospitals were required to provide free or below-cost medical services. The 1913 legislation was reinforced in 1956 by the passage of a revenue ruling specifying that "a hospital was charitable only if it operated to the extent of its financial ability for those not able to pay for the services rendered and not exclusively for those able and expected to pay."[45] Private not-for-profit hospitals remain the largest hospital sector; they currently account for 60 percent of all U.S. acute care hospitals. The number of beds in this sector increased by 28 percent in the decade following the passage of the 1965 Medicare and Medicaid legislation.

Because of the legislation noted above, a hospital had to provide free or below-cost care to those unable to pay in order to retain its not-for-profit status. This situation changed in 1969 when the Revenue Ruling superseded the 1956 and 1913 legislation, requiring merely that not-for-profit hospitals provide services that benefit the community.[46] The authors of the 1969 revenue ruling conjectured that the Medicare and Medicaid legislation passed in 1965 would eliminate the need for hospital charitable care.[47] These policy makers believed that the newly passed Medicare and Medicaid legislation would guarantee health-care coverage for everyone.[48] Finally, these lawmakers also believed hospitals should provide more to the community than simply charitable care.

Following passage of the 1969 legislation, hospital administrators assessed the demand for charitable care in a new light. Not-for-profit hospitals were freed from the burden of caring for the poor; these hospitals could now retain their tax-exempt status by providing health care to the community as a whole. The vagueness of this requirement prompted a wide variety of responses under the guise of providing health care to the community.[49] For example, many not-for-profit hospitals maintained their tax-exempt status by investing in high-tech equipment and new buildings "for the sake of the community." As a result, not-for-profit hospitals became a "converging point for highly skilled professionals and their supporting technicians."[50] One analyst described this emerging strategy among not-for-profit hospitals as "the medical arms race."[51] Because this legislation enabled many not-for-profit hospitals to behave like their for-profit counterparts, many researchers claim that it led to a narrowing of the distinction between not-for-profit and for-profit hospitals.[52]

Researchers and community representatives indicate that many not-for-profit hospitals have not been meeting the needs of their communities.[53] The actions of three state governments illustrate this dissatisfaction.[54] Recently Texas, Utah and Vermont have tried to standardize the qualifications that not-for-profit hospitals must meet in order to maintain their not-for-profit status. Texas— the first state to hold non-profit hospitals accountable for their tax-exempt status—compares the dollar amount of charity care provided by not-for-profit hospitals with their estimated tax benefits.[55] Hospitals that do not provide charity care equal in value to their estimated tax benefits are required to pay state fines. For instance, a not-for-profit Texas hospital was required to pay penalties after receiving an estimated $44 million dollars in tax benefits while providing only $8 million dollars in charity care.[56] Utah determines a hospital's not-for-profit status based on its prior-year contributions to the community: "Considerable attention is paid to the . . . dollar amount of free or uncompensated care provided to the local population. In effect, if that amount exceeds what would have been the property tax, the hospital's property is tax exempt."[57] Vermont's approach to the determination of a hospital's not-for-profit status is slightly different than Utah's: Vermont tests the availability of charity care at the not-for-profit hospital rather than the hospital's actual quantified gift to the community.[58] Policy makers and administrators continue to debate the level of charity care required for not-for-profit hospitals to retain their exempt status. Meanwhile government not-for-profit hospitals treat a higher proportion of uninsured patients than private not-for-profit hospitals.

The government not-for-profit hospital sector. Since the 1700s, governmental not-for-profit hospitals (public hospitals) have played a vivid role in the history of American hospitals. Many big-city public hospitals began as almshouses, including Bellevue in New York, Charity in New Orleans and Cook County in Chicago. In 1902, government not-for-profit hospitals were described as grim and barracks-like; they typically had wards for patients with syphilis, tuberculosis and mental disorders and for unmarried pregnant women.[59]

Policy makers predicted the closure of many government not-for-profit hospitals following passage of the 1965 Medicare and Medicaid legislation, which gave the poor the means to pay for hospital care.[60] "In theory, all patients now were paying patients and were entitled to private care."[61] This prediction did not come true, and a mass closing of government not-for-profit hospitals never occurred. Government not-for-profit hospitals currently account for 26 percent of all U.S. acute care hospitals.[62]

Government not-for-profit hospitals are an important component in the not-for-profit/for-profit hospital debate. The presence of government hospitals in a community influences the strategies of the other hospitals, both for-profit and private not-for-profit. Research indicates that government not-for-profit hospitals often care for patients that other hospitals consider undesirable. A disproportionate number of their patients are poor, uninsured or Medicaid recipients.[63]

Some researchers question whether the care at government not-for-profit hospitals is comparable to care at their private not-for-profit and for-profit counterparts. For example, researchers who recently compared the records of patients suffering from ischemic heart disease at the three types of hospitals found that patients at government not-for-profit hospitals received less extensive services than patients at for-profit and private not-for-profit hospitals. Likewise, other researchers find that patients at government not-for-profit hospitals received fewer diagnostic tests, fewer surgeries, and fewer follow-up visits.[64]

The For-Profit Hospital Sector

Historically, the for-profit hospital sector has had a large role in the American health care industry. In the early 1900s, many for-profit hospitals were operated by physicians in rural areas where other types of hospitals were nonexistent. In urban areas, eminent surgeons opened for-profit hospitals for patients who preferred not to seek treatment at not-for-profit hospitals.[65] In 1910, for-profit hospitals accounted for approximately 50 percent of all hospitals, out of 4,000 hospitals in 1910, 1,500 to 2,000 were for-profit hospitals.[66] Thereafter, the number of proprietary hospitals steadily decreased as "community hospitals opened their staffs to wider membership and doctors found that they were able to have the public provide the capital for hospitals and maximize their incomes through professional fees."[67] By 1928, according to Starr, proprietary hospitals accounted for only 36 percent of all hospitals. The number of proprietary hospitals subsequently declined further, to 27 percent and then 18 percent of all hospitals, in 1938 and 1946, respectively.

The for-profit sector experienced unprecedented growth following the passage of the 1965 federal Medicare and Medicaid legislation. This legislation was responsible for an infusion of dollars into the health-care industry. Although for-profit hospitals accounted for 15 percent of all short-term general hospitals in 1965 and today account for 11 percent, the number of beds in the for-profit sector grew by 55 percent, from 47,000 to 73,000 beds in the decade following the passage of this legislation.[68] In 1990, the American Hospital Federation reported that the twenty largest for-profit hospital chains owned over 80 percent of these for-profit hospitals.

Research indicates that these chains avoid locating in states with strong hospital regulatory systems.[69] Proprietary chains also avoid states with mandatory price-control programs. Researchers found that only 3 percent of proprietary hospital chains' revenue was subject to mandatory rate review.[70]

For-profit chains also consider economic conditions in their location decisions. Research indicates that for-profit hospitals choose to locate in affluent areas, purposely avoiding the provision of expensive charitable care that detracts from potential hospital profits.[71] For-profit hospitals also avoid high-cost, low-profit services like outpatient departments, emergency-rooms and teaching programs.[72]

The darlings of Wall Street, for-profit hospital stocks have earned record returns for their investors. Critics indicate, however, that these record returns are not always gains for their communities. Potential stockholders do not base their purchasing decisions on how well the hospitals are meeting community needs.[73] Furthermore, a for-profit hospital's interest in community welfare is demonstrably weaker if the hospital is affiliated with a for-profit chain.[74]

Table 1 presents a breakdown by type of all U.S. hospitals in each of the years covered by this research (see Chapter 3 for an explanation of the data source).

If, as researchers postulate, the distinction between for-profit and not-for-profit hospitals is narrowing, what phenomena should we be able to observe? First, we should expect not-for-profit hospitals to cut their costs, by such means as shortening their average lengths of stay or cutting their medical staffs. We would also expect

Table 1. Number of U.S. hospitals by type and year

hospital profit status:	1980 number (% total)	1985 number (% total)	1990 number (% total)	1994 number (% total)
for-profit	557	622	594	491
	(11%)	(12%)	(12%)	(11%)
private not-for-profit	2368	2421	2314	2181
	(46%)	(47%)	(48%)	(50%)
religious not-for-profit	671	654	601	528
	(13%)	(13%)	(12%)	(12%)
government not-for-profit	1537	1439	1338	1196
	(30%)	(28%)	(28%)	(27%)
Total N	5133	5136	4847	4396

not-for-profit hospitals to reduce their provision of community service. For example, we could expect not-for-profit hospitals to reduce their provision of emergency services or close their emergency departments. Additionally, we could expect not-for-profit hospitals to eliminate some of their unprofitable outpatient services, including immunizations and screenings. Simply put, if what Starr and other researchers argue is true, it should become increasingly difficult to distinguish a not-for-profit hospital from a for-profit hospital. The remainder of this chapter uses neo-institutional theory to analyze the hypothesis of a narrowing distinction between hospital types.

EXPLANATIONS FOR THE HYPOTHETICAL CONVERGENCE OF HOSPITAL TYPES

If the distinction between not-for-profit and for-profit hospitals is narrowing, what explains their convergence? Neo-institutional theory illustrates how environmental factors tend to blur distinctions between organizational types. Neo-institutionalists have repeatedly demonstrated that firms' strategies are predicated on existing public policy. Put simply, policy establishes the rules regarding (1) how firms may organize (e.g., charter laws), (2) how firms deal with wealth (e.g., tax laws), (3) what assets firms can exploit for profit (i.e., policy rights), (4) how firms deal with employees (e.g., affirmative action) and (5) how firms deal with competitors (e.g., antitrust laws). Given the constitutive role of policy, it is not surprising that new policies often spur drastic industry-wide change, prompting organizations to adopt new strategies.[75] Neo-institutionalists also argue that attention to policy helps us understand the timing of the complex responses that follow in its wake.

Significant Federal Policy

Neo-institutionalists hypothesize that new legislation in an organization's environment increases the likelihood that isomorphism (declining differences between organizational types) will occur. Recent research confirms that changes in the regulatory environment affect hospital outcomes. For example, Duffy and Farley find that hospitals may discontinue inpatient procedures as a result of changes in the regulatory environment. "[U]sing data from the

Agency for Health Care Policy and Research's Healthcare Cost and Utilization Project, . . . [they] studied the 150 procedures that were most frequently performed on inpatients in 1980. They found that (a) 37 of the 150 procedures declined in use more than 40 percent by 1987, (b) patients that continued to receive one of the 37 procedures in 1987 on an inpatient basis tended to be more severely ill than in 1980, and (c) rates of decline were disproportionately large for Medicaid recipients."[76]

These findings enable neo-institutionalists to expand on neo-classical economic explanations by demonstrating that current policy influences organizational responses to local demand and supply conditions. Therefore, neo-institutionalists postulate that hospital personnel's responses to demand and supply are not solely dependent on local conditions. Instead, hospital administrators review current policy as they develop strategies for managing local demand and supply. Neo-institutionalists argue that organizational outcomes converge as the personnel of separate organizations adopt similar strategies to comply with regulatory changes. Fligstein demonstrates that the largest U.S. firms have been forced to change their dominant strategies following the passage of federal legislation. Prior to passage of anti-cartel legislation in the 1920s, the dominant strategy of large firms revolved around attempts to control markets. Similarly, the passage of the Celler Kefauver Act in 1950 prohibited firms from using horizontal and vertical integration as means of expansion.[77]

The implementation of the Medicare Prospective Payment System (PPS) in 1983 is the most significant health-care policy enacted in the past twenty-five years. The purpose of the Medicare Prospective Payment System legislation is to regulate Medicare reimbursement. The Prospective Payment System marked the beginning of the use of price controls at the national level in the hospital industry.[78] In a sense, the implementation of PPS changed the rules of the game. Therefore, let us look at whether the hospital industry's response to PPS is consistent with the findings of past neo-institutional research.

Enactment of the Prospective Payment System

With the passage of the Prospective Payment System, in 1983, the hospital industry was faced with cost-containment legislation for the first time in its history. Previously, hospitals had used their own discretion in pricing hospital services.[79] The Prospective Payment System legislation eliminated such discretion by authorizing the government to establish uniform prices for all hospital services for Medicare patients. Furthermore, the Prospective Payment System legislation changed the incentive structure in the hospital industry. In fact, many researchers pointed out "the need for non-profit hospitals to act like businesses because of the scaled-back Medicare payment."[80]

The Prospective Payment System uses Diagnostic Related Groups (DRGs) to determine the payment for each medical treatment.[81] Specifically, the record of each Medicare-eligible patient is coded with a DRG before the patient leaves the hospital. DRGs determine all Medicare reimbursements paid to hospitals.[82] Because the legislation mandated that all hospitals receive the same reimbursements for treating Medicare patients, reimbursement is the same for identical treatment at a for-profit and a not-for-profit hospital. Therefore, the PPS legislation forced both not-for-profit and for-profit hospitals to closely monitor their costs to ensure that Medicare reimbursements covered their costs for Medicare patients. In other words the PPS legislation required all not-for-profit and for-profit hospitals to accept established price controls. Therefore, hospitals were forced to incur costs lower than the reimbursement amount to make a profit. "PPS was a fixed payment per case determined in advance . . . this approach offered hospitals the rewards of a profit or the penalty of a loss."[83]

The example of a 68 year old man with Medicare insurance undergoing coronary-bypass surgery illustrates this change. Prior to implementation of the Prospective Payment System, a hospital had every incentive to keep the coronary-bypass surgery patient in the hospital for a few extra days following his surgery. The hospital also had an incentive to perform supplementary pre-operative and post-operative tests. The hospital would have been reimbursed for all or almost all of the costs of caring for the patient. However, if the same man had coronary-bypass surgery in 1985, following implementation of the PPS, the hospital would have every incentive to provide less care. It might well release the patient earlier and perform fewer pre- and post-operative tests than in the days prior to passage of the Prospective Payment System.

Following passage of the PPS, the government mandated that it would reimburse the hospital a standard amount for medical procedures. If the reimbursement amount for coronary-bypass surgery was $15,000 and it only cost the hospital $11,000 to perform surgery on the patient, the hospital made a $4,000 profit. But if the patient had medical complications or the procedure was delayed, and it ended up costing the hospital $20,000 to treat the patient, the hospital lost $5,000.

In a study of intensive-care admissions in one medical center hospital, researchers found that, in some cases, a stable Medicare patient was transferred from a regular hospital ward to the intensive-care unit. This move enabled the hospital to increase revenues by $500 with considerably smaller increases in cost. However, Medicare reimbursements for some of the sickest patients in the intensive-care unit, including those who had undergone coronary-bypass surgery, were barely more than half of actual treatment costs.[84]

It is important to point out that most hospitals did not know their costs for a given procedure in 1983. For the most part, hospitals still did not know the cost of a given procedure in 1994. However, hospitals do know their annual aggregate expenses, which are compiled for income statements by their auditors. These aggregated audited numbers are the figures used in this research. This phenomenon is consistent with neo-institutional theorists who indicate that there is a decoupling between an organization's core (in this case the expenses/money) and the actual hospital structure.[85]

Health policy prior to the implementation of PPS was prescriptive; it provided instruction for hospitals on how to meet its requirements. It is important to recognize that the PPS legislation was the first time that hospitals were given conditions to meet, yet without instructions on how they were supposed to do business under this new capitated system.

For instance, the Hill Burton Act (1945)—a partnership between voluntary hospitals and the states—provided federal money to build hospitals and improve existing structures. "For the first time, the federal government became an important force in sustaining the hospital as a local institution, through direct subsidy (via the Hill-Burton program of federal grants to states) and through federal tax incentives."[86] The Hill Burton Act specified how this money was to be spent, as well as other criteria. Similarly, the 1965 passage of Medicare and Medicaid also gave money to hospitals, once again with precise guidelines; the federal government would reimburse hospitals for treating patients age sixty-five and over and patients with Medicaid insurance. The 1969 Internal Revenue Service Ruling enlarged not-for-profit hospitals' definition of charitable care, giving hospitals more leeway in maintaining their exemption status. In each of these cases, hospitals were told exactly how to meet the demands of this new legislation. Following passage of the Prospective Payment System, by contrast, hospitals were forced to accept price controls, but given no instruction on how to work under these price controls. This was the first time hospitals were faced with proscriptive rather than prescriptive legislation.

Organizations experiment with a variety of strategies to meet new legislative mandates. During the current period of experimentation, organizations are carefully monitoring the strategies of other organizations in their environments and looking to each other for ideas. Not-for-profit and for-profit hospitals are likely to look to each other to make sense out of the new cost-containment legislation.

Neo-institutionalists explain that organizations mimic the behavior of other organizations they perceive to be successful.[87] In the five years prior to passage of this legislation, policymakers had become alarmed at rising health-care costs. Therefore, the hospitals perceived as successful were those with low operating costs. Other hospitals began to mimic the strategies and behaviors of hospitals that were appropriately managing their costs. The widespread adoption of cost-saving strategies could be attributed to a declining distinction between hospital types. Hospitals can also be expected to alter their strategies to align with the policy changes in order to achieve their goals. DiMaggio and Powell indicate that increased regulatory constraints force organizations to adopt similar strategies that result in similar outcomes.

As we have just seen, the PPS legislation forced both not-for-profit and for-profit hospitals to work under established price controls. This constraint forced hospitals to incur costs lower than the Medicare reimbursement amount in order to keep their income statements in the black. This situation generates two hypotheses:

Hypotheses 1: Over the past fifteen years, all things being equal, there has been a convergence in the nation's short-term general hospitals as measured by efficiency and community-service outcomes.

More specifically, the impact of type of ownership decreases as organizations adopt similar strategies.

> Hypotheses 1a: As financial risk in the health-care industry increases, hospital type (private not-for-profit, religious not-for-profit, government not-for-profit and for-profit) becomes less significant in explaining differences between individual hospitals in efficiency and community-service outcomes in recent years compared with previous years.

Alternative Policy Explanations

Others have found that this cost-saving legislation had opposite effects of what the PPS legislation intended. Researchers argue that the Prospective Payment System legislation increased profits for both for-profit and not-for-profit hospitals.[88] They assert that the cost ceilings implemented by the Prospective Payment System were more lucrative than the previous payment structure. If they are correct, one could speculate that this legislation enabled hospitals to spend more money to develop programs that met the needs of their administrators, medical staff and communities. If so, this legislation increased hospital freedom and did not constrain existing freedoms. Therefore we may expect no subsequent blurring of the distinction between hospital types.

Alternatively, one could argue that this legislation did not result in cost savings but in rising costs. Following passage of the Prospective Payment System legislation, hospitals could no longer rely on accounting clerks and a manual or antiquated computer system. Instead hospitals needed more sophisticated cost-accounting measures. Therefore, one could hypothesize that they hired savvy financial and accounting personnel who demanded higher salaries than had the former accounting clerks. Additionally, hospitals may have installed sophisticated computer systems to track appropriate cost information. Therefore, one could expect that increases in the cost of the accounting staff as well as sophisticated computer systems would increase the total expenses per adjusted admission at the not-for-profit hospitals. In other words, the cost-containment legislation became a cost burden for private not-for-profit hospitals.

Since for-profit hospitals historically have had a reputation for controlling and monitoring costs, one could conclude that this legislation was not a financial burden for them. Therefore, in this scenario one may expect that the PPS legislation will increase expenses per adjusted admission at the not-for-profit hospitals, resulting in a sharper distinction between not-for-profit and for-profit hospitals, rather than a less sharp distinction.

For example, one may hypothesize that the Prospective Payment System legislation moved the accounting department from the back offices to the front lines, and that many more hospital administrators with accounting and finance backgrounds were hired following implementation of this legislation. Fligstein demonstrates that legislative changes dictate the backgrounds of chief executive officers in Fortune 100 companies.[89] The hiring of more administrators with backgrounds in accounting and finance would tend to make hospitals more cost-conscious than they had been in the past. Furthermore, many of these accounting and finance personnel are likely to have been trained at similar programs and to be members of the same professional organizations.

Alternative Explanations Other Than Policy

Many other factors besides policy could be used to explain the hypothesized convergence in the hospital industry. For instance, one could invoke similar internal characteristics, such as the affiliation of increasing numbers of both types of hospitals with hospital systems, or a narrowing of the size difference between for-profit and not-for-profit hospitals over the past fifteen years. Another possible explanation is that not-for-profit hospitals are reducing their commitment to teaching. Or one could invoke growing similarities between not-for-profit and for-profit hospital case mixes. Finally, it could be argued that as both types of hospitals continue to increase their investments in technology, reduce lengths of stay and substitute lower skilled licensed practical nurses for higher skilled registered nurses, the distinction between for-profit and not-for-profit hospitals will decline.

Environmental explanations include competition at the local level and regulation at the state level. Other external factors might be a high ratio of specialist MDs to generalist MDs, or a high proportion of HMO members in the local population. Finally, a changing demographic profile of potential hospital clients could be explanatory if, for instance, the proportion of the local population over the age of sixty-five were increasing, or if a change in average per-capita income resulted from the opening or closing of a large employer.

In the present analysis of the relationship between hospital ownership type and hospital community service and efficiency outcomes, the research controls for internal and environmental factors used in previous research. In Chapter 4, these factors are discussed in greater detail.

SUMMARY

This chapter describes neo-institutional theory, the theoretical framework, of this research, and explains why the hospital industry is a good test case of its merits. Additionally, the chapter traces the analytical and historical distinction between for-profit and not-for-profit hospitals, and provides a description of what we can expect to happen if the distinction between not-for-profit and for-profit hospital outcomes has in fact declined. After describing in detail the new policy, the 1983 Prospective Payment System, that forced hospitals to develop new strategies, the chapter explores a variety of alternative explanations. The next two chapters describe how the claims of a declining distinction between hospital types were examined. Chapter 3 describes in detail the data and dependent variables used in this analysis. Chapter 4 discusses the organizational and environmental factors (independent variables) that were controlled for in this analysis.

NOTES

1. See P. J. DiMaggio, and W. W. Powell, "The Iron Cage Revisited: Institutional Isomorphism and Collective Rationality in Organizational Fields," *American Sociological Review* 48 (1983) 147–60; N. Fligstein, "The Spread of the Multidivsional Firm, 1919–79," *American Sociological Review* 501 (1985) 377–391; N. Fligstein, "The Intraorganizational Power Struggle: Rise of Finance Personnel to Top Leadership in Large Corporations, 1919–1979," *American Sociological Review* 52 (1987) 44–58.

2. Philip Selznick, *TVA and the Grass Roots* (New York: Harper and Row, 1965).

3.   Charles Perrow, *Complex Organizations: A Critical Essay* (New York: McGraw-Hill, 1986).

4.   See Paul R. Lawrence, and Jay W. Lorsch, *Organization and Environment* (Cambridge, Massachusetts: Harvard University Press, 1967); Perrow, *Complex Organizations;* James Thompson, *Organizations in Action* (New York: McGraw-Hill, 1967).

5.   S. Strasser, "The Effective Application of Contingency Theory in Health Settings: Problems and Recommended Solutions," *Health Care Management Review.* Winter (1983). 15–23; S. M. Shortell, and A. D. Kaluzny. "Organization Theory and Health Services Management," in *Health Care Management.* ed. S. M. Shortell, and A. D. Kaluzny, Albany, New York: Delmar Publishers, 1994) 3–29.

6.   Shortell, and Kaluzny, "Organization Theory and Health Services Management."

7.   Jeffrey Pfeffer, and Gerald Salanzick, *The External Control of Organizations* (New York: Harper and Row, 1978).

8.   J. A. Alexander, A. S. Kaluzny, and S. C. Middleton, "Organizational Growth, Survival and Death in the U.S. Hospital Industry: A Population Ecology Perspective," *Social Science and Medicine* 22 (1986): 304.

9.   Ibid., 305.

10.   M. T. Hannan, and J. H. Freeman. "The Population Ecology of Organizations," *American Journal of Sociology* 82 (1977): 929–64.

11.   W. Richard Scott, *Organizations: Rational, Natural and Open Systems* (Englewood Cliffs, NJ: Prentice-Hall, 1987).

12.   Shortell, and Kaluzny. "Organization Theory and Health Services Management."

13.   Selznick, *TVA and the Grass Roots.*

14.   DiMaggio and Powell "The Iron Cage Revisited."

15.   Edward O. Laumann, Joseph. Galaskiewicz, and Peter Marsden, "Community Structure as Interorganizational Linkage," *Annual Review of Sociology* 4 (1978): 455–84. 1978; DiMaggio and Powell "The Iron Cage Revisited."

16.   DiMaggio and Powell "The Iron Cage Revisited."

17.   Ibid., 150

18.   N. Fligstein, "The Spread of the Multidivsional Firm;" N. Fligstein, "The Structural Transformation of American Industry: An Institutional Account of the Causes of Diversification in the Largest Firms, 1919–1979," In *The New Institutionalism in Organizational Analysis,* ed. W. W. Powell and P. J. DiMaggio, (Chicago: The University of Chicago Press, 1991): 311–336.

19.   C. L. Estes, and J.H. Swan, "Privatization, System Membership and Access to Home Health Care for the Elderly," *Milbank Quarterly* 72 (1994): 277–298.

20.   J. N. Baron, F. R. Dobbin, and P. D. Jennings, "War and Peace: The Evolution of Modern Personnel Administration in U.S. Industry," *American Journal of Sociology* 92 (1986): 350–383.

21.   See N. Fligstein, "The Spread of the Multidivsional Firm;" N. Fligstein, "The Structural Transformation of American Industry;" F. Dobbin, and T. J. Dowd. "How Policy Shapes Competition: Early Railroad Foundings in Massachusetts," *Administrative Science Quarterly* 42 (1997): 501–529.

22.   Cheryl I. Hultman, "Uncompensated Care before and after Prospective Payment: The Role of Hospital Location and Ownership," *Health Services Research* 26 (1991): 614–22.

23.   DiMaggio and Powell "The Iron Cage Revisited," 151.

24.   B. Levit, B. and C. Nass. "The Lid on the Garbage Can: Institutional Constraints on Decision Making in the Technical Core of College-Text Publishers," *Administrative Science Quarterly* 34 (1989): 190–207.

25.   See P. S., Tolbert and L. G. Zucker, "Institutional Sources of Change in the Formal Structure of Organizations: The Diffusion of Civil Service Reform, 1880–1935," *Administrative Science Quarterly* 28 (1983): 22–39.

26.   R. Kuttner, "Columbia/HCA and the Resurgence of the For-Profit Hospital Business," *New England Journal of Medicine* 335 (1996): 446–51.

27.   S. Woolhandler, and D. U. Himmelstein. "Costs of care and administration at for-profit and other hospitals in the United States," *The New England Journal of Medicine* 336 (1997): 773.

28.   B. Arrington, and C. C. Haddock, "Who Really Profits from Not-For-Profits?" *Health Services Research* 25 (1990): 291–304.

29.   DiMaggio and Powell "The Iron Cage Revisited."

30.   Ibid., 152.

31.   P. J. DiMaggio, "Constructing an Organizational Field as a Professional Project," In *The New Institutionalism in Organizational Analysis*, ed. W. W. Powell and P. J. DiMaggio, (Chicago: The University of Chicago Press, 1991), 267–292.

32.   Ibid.

33.   Rosemary Stevens, *In Sickness and In Wealth.*:

34.   Ibid.

35.   John W Meyer, and Brian Rowan. "Institutionalized Organizations: Formal Structure as Myth and Ceremony," *American Journal of Sociology* 83 (1977): 364–385; DiMaggio and Powell "The Iron Cage Revisited."

36.   C. G. Homer, D. D. Bradham, and M. Rushefsky. "To the Editor, Investor-Owned and Not-For-Profit Hospitals: Beyond the Cost and Revenue Debate," *Health Affairs* (1984): 133–136.

37.   Bradford H. Gray, *The Profit Motive and Patient Care: The Changing Accountability of Doctors and Hospitals* (Cambridge, Massachusetts: Harvard University Press, 1991), 22.

38.   Ibid., 61.

39.   William A. Rushing, "Profit and Nonprofit Orientations and the Differentiations-Coordination Hypothesis for Organizations: A Study of Small General Hospitals," *American Sociological Review* 41 (1976): 676–91.

40.   Ibid.

41.   See also Henry Hansman, "The Role of Nonprofit Enterprise," *Yale Law Journal* 89 (1980): 835–901; P. J. DiMaggio, "Support for the Arts from Private Foundations," in *Nonprofit Enterprise in the Arts*, ed. P. J. DiMaggio, (New York: Oxford University Press, 1986), 113–39.

42.   M. J. Vogel, "The Invention of the Modern Hospitals: Boston, 1879–1930," Chicago: University of Chicago Press, 1980), 127.

43.   J. Mann, G. Melnick, A. Bamezai, and J. Zwanziger. "Uncompensated Care: Hospitals' Responses to Fiscal Pressures," *Health Affairs* (1995): 236–270.

44.   Rosemary Stevens, *In Sickness and In Wealth.*

45.   D. M. Fox, and D. C. Schaffer. "Tax Administration as Health Policy: Hospitals, the Internal Revenue Service and the Courts," *Journal of Health Politics, Policy and Law* 16 (1991): 257.

46.   D. M. Fox, and D. C. Schaffer. "Tax Administration as Health Policy: Hospitals, the Internal Revenue Service and the Courts," *Journal of Health Politics, Policy and Law* 16 (1991): 251–279.

47.   Ibid.

48.   Ibid.

49.   Ibid.

50.   Ibid., 262.

51.   Nancy Kane, "Report on the Financial Resources of Major Hospitals in Boston." (Boston: Department of Health and Hospitals, 1993).

52.   Fox, and Schaffer. "Tax Administration as Health Policy;" H. P. Tuckman and C. Y. Chang. "A Proposal to Redistribute the Cost of Hospital Charity Care," *The Milbank Quarterly* 69 (1991): 113–141.

53.   see Nancy Kane, "Report on the Financial Resources of Major Hospitals in Boston."

54.   J. W. O'Donnel, and J. H. Taylor. "The Bounds of Charity; the Current Status of the Hospital Property-Tax exemption," *The New England*

Journal of Medicine 322 (1990): 65–67; M. Jee, "Texas Links Charity Care, Hospital Tax-Exempt Status," *Journal of American Health Policy* 3 (1993).

55. M. Jee, "Texas Links Charity Care, Hospital Tax-Exempt Status," *Journal of American Health Policy* 3 (1993).

56. Ibid.

57. O'Donnel, and Taylor. "The Bounds of Charity," 66.

58. O'Donnel, and Taylor. "The Bounds of Charity."

59. Rosemary Stevens, *In Sickness and In Wealth.*

60. Fox, and Schaffer. "Tax Administration as Health Policy;" F. W. Blaisdell, "Development of the City-County Public Hospital," *Archives of Surgery* 129 (1994): 760–764.

61. Blaisdell, "Development of the City-County Public Hospital."

62. American Hospital Association. *1992 AHA Guide* (Chicago: American Hospital Association, 1992).

63. E. Brown, "Public Hospitals on the Brink: Their Problems and Their Options," *Journal of Health Politics, Policy and Law* 7(1983): 928.

64. M. J. Yedidia, "Differences in Treatment of Ischemic Heart Disease at a Public and a Voluntary Hospital: Sources and Consequences," *The Milbank Quarterly* 72 (1994): 299–327.

65. Rosemary Stevens, *In Sickness and In Wealth.*

66. Ibid.

67. Paul Starr, *The Social Transformation of American Medicine* (New York: Basic Books, 1982), 219.

68. E. Ginzberg, "For-Profit Medicine: A Reassessment," *New England Journal of Medicine* 319 (1988): 757–61; American Hospital Association. *The AHA Profile of Hospital Statistics* (Chicago: American Hospital Association, 1993/94).

69. E. Ginzberg, "For-Profit Medicine: A Reassessment."

70. Edmund R. Becker, and Frank Sloan. "Hospital Ownership and Performance," *Economic Inquiry* 23 (1985): 21–35.

71. E. C. Norton, and D. O. Staiger. "How Hospitals Ownership Affects Access to Care for the Uninsured," *Rand Journal of Economics* 25 (1994): 171–85.

72. E. Ginzberg, "For-Profit Medicine: A Reassessment."

73. Rushing, "Profit and Nonprofit Orientations."

74. Ibid.

75. Fligstein, "The Intraorganizational Power Struggle;" Fligstein, "The Structural Transformation of American Industry;" F. Dobbin, J. R. Sutton, J. W. Meyer. and W. R. Scott. "Equal Opportunity and the Construction of Internal Labor Markets," *American Journal of Sociology* 99

(1993): 396–427; F. Dobbin, and T. J. Dowd "How Policy Shapes Competition: Early Railroad Foundings in Massachusetts," *Administrative Science Quarterly* 42 (1997): 501–529.

76.   Sarah Q. Duffy, and Dean E. Farley, "Patterns of Decline among Inpatient Procedures," *Public Health Reports* 110 (1995): 674–681.

77.   Fligstein (1991)

78.   Different states experimented with hospital price controls prior to the passage of PPS. These states include Connecticut (1974), Maryland (1973), Massachusetts (1971), New Jersey (1971), New York (1969), Rhode Island (1971), Washington (1973), and Wisconsin (1975). See Charles E. Phelps, *Health Economics* (New York: Harper Collins Publishers, 1990), 474.

79.   Until 1982, most hospitals had their own billing systems and their own billing forms. The 1982 UB82 legislation standardized the billing system in all United States hospitals by mandating that all hospitals use the UB82 form for all hospital billings. The legislation forced both not-for-profit and for-profit hospitals to reorganize their finance, accounting and computer departments in an effort to track the needed information. Before the UB82 legislation, there was no single, standard method of tracking hospital costs. Following its passage, hospitals could compare their own performance to that of their not-for-profit and for-profit counterparts.

80.   E. A. Sorrentino, "Hospital Mission and Cost Differences," *Hospital Topics* 67 1989: 22; M. Waldholdtz, "To Keep Doors Open, Non-profits Act Like Businesses," *The Wall Street Journal*, (December 12, 1982); D. Coddington, L. Palmquist, and W. Trollinger. "Strategies for Survival in the Hospital Industry," *Harvard Business Review* May–June (1985): 129–38.

81.   Approximately 467 DRGs represent a clustering of diseases that are likely to affect those who are eligible for Medicare. The DRGs are based upon the *9000 International Classification of Diseases*. DRGs are the product produced by the hospital, and they do not take into consideration case-mix severity. For example, DRG 103 designates a heart transplant. See for explanation, Rosemary Stevens, *In Sickness and In Wealth.*

82.   Rosemary Stevens, *In Sickness and In Wealth.*

83.   S. H. Altman, and D. A. Young. "A Decade of Medicare's Prospective Payment System—Success or Failure?" *Journal of American Health Policy.* March/April (1993): 12.

84.   D. P. Wagner, T. D. Wineland, and W. A. Knaus. "The Hidden Costs of Treating Severely Ill Patients: Charges and resource consumption in an intensive care unit," *Health Care Financing Review* 5 (1983): 81–86.

85.   John W. Meyer, and Richard W. Scott. 1983. *Organizational Environments: Ritual and Rationality* (Beverly Hills, California: Sage, 1983).

86. Rosemary Stevens, *In Sickness and In Wealth,* 228.

87. T. J. Dowd, and F. Dobbin. "Was There a Market Before Antitrust?: Public Policy and Railroad Strategy in Early America," in *Constructing Markets and Industries,* ed. J. Porac and M. Ventresa, Forthcoming. (New York: Pergamon Press, 1998).

88. Chang and Tuckman. "The Profits of Not-For-Profit Hospitals," *Journal of Health Politics, Policy and Law* 13 (1988): 547–64.

89. Fligstein, "The Intraorganizational Power Struggle."

CHAPTER 3

Indices of Hospital Performance

This chapter describes the data used to assess the claims of a narrowing distinction between hospital types. If these claims are correct, the efficiency and community-service outcomes of these two types of hospitals will tend to converge over time.

DATA

The analysis utilizes secondary data from the American Hospital Association and data from the Area Resource Files. The American Hospital Association compiles data from virtually every hospital in the United States; the Area Resource File provides demographic data for each of the 3248 counties in the contiguous United States. Linking internal hospital data from the American Hospital Association with county-level data from the Area Resource File enabled the researcher to analyze the claims of a declining distinction between hospital types in light of data about the hospitals' local environments.

American Hospital Association Data

The American Hospital Association (AHA) surveys every hospital in the country annually. Data were obtained on all short-term general hospitals in the contiguous United States—which are self-identified in the following categories: for-profit, private not-for-profit, religious not-for-profit and government not-for-profit. Moreover, these data were utilized at four- to five-year intervals

(1980, 1985, 1990, 1994)—for the fifteen year period 1980–1994. The American Hospital Association defines acute-care hospitals as "general medical and surgical hospitals" in which the "average length of stay for all patients is less than 30 days or over 50 percent of all patients are admitted to units where the average length of stay is less than 30 days." Such hospitals are distinguished from mental-health and specialty hospitals.[1]

The American Hospital Association survey contains missing data, as hospitals do not always provide information on every question. The Health Care Information Resources Group of the American Hospital Association—which uses these data to compile annual data bases, hospital directories and hospital statistics—interpolates or extrapolates data for hospitals that do not complete the survey. Non responsive hospitals numbered 555 in 1980, 424 in 1985, 321 in 1990 and 527 in 1994. Hospitals for which data were interpolated or extrapolated were excluded in order to avoid the ambiguity that the use of such data can introduce.[2]

Area Resource File Data

The Area Resource Files compiled annually by the Bureau of Health Professions contain environmental and demographic data on the 3,248 counties in the contiguous United States. These 3,248 counties remain the same across the 15 years in the study.

Linking the American Hospital Association data and the Area Resource File data enabled the researcher to derive an accurate picture of hospitals and their environments, and to draw sound conclusions about the prospects of a narrowing distinction between not-for-profit and for-profit hospitals. Chapter 5 explains the methods used to link the two data sources.

HOSPITAL OUTCOMES

Other researchers have used similarities in hospital outcomes to demonstrate a convergence between for-profit and not-for-profit hospitals.[3] This research uses both efficiency and community-service outcomes. For each category of outcomes, two dependent variables were chosen which were used in prior research. The two dependent variables used as a proxy for efficiency are total hospital expense per adjusted admission and the number of full-time-equivalent employees per adjusted census. For provision of community service, the two variables are emergency-room visits per adjusted inpatient day and outpatient visits per adjusted inpatient day. *Table 2* presents the means and standard deviations for the dependent variables for each year in the study.

Efficiency Outcomes

Historically, researchers have linked efficiency outcomes and hospital ownership type. More specifically, they have examined the efficiency of for-profit hospitals. Because for-profit hospitals distribute their profits to owners or shareholders, for-profit hospitals are often viewed as moneymaking agencies susceptible to the vigorous scrutiny of return-conscious investors and owners. This view has led to the assumption that for-profit hospitals are more efficient than their not-for-profit counterparts. In recent years, however, many researchers have argued that the cost-conscious focus of the Prospective Payment System has forced not-for-profit hospitals, like their for-profit counterparts, to focus on cost-saving strategies in an effort to become more efficient. Two of the most visible efficiency strategies are reducing hospital costs and reducing the size of the hospital medical staff. Therefore, the total hospital expenses per adjusted admission and the number of full-time-equivalents per adjusted census were used as proxies for hospital efficiency.

Total Hospital Expense per Adjusted Admission

Definition. Total hospital expense per adjusted admission is an accepted proxy for hospital efficiency.[4] Total hospital expenses are the annual costs incurred to operate the hospital. In other words, all costs that contribute to the daily operation of the hospital are referred to as hospital expenses. Examples include payroll expenses, administration and billing, cafeteria, medical supplies, operating-room expenses and hospital lab expenses. Costs incurred in the construction of a new hospital wing or the purchase of new high-tech equipment are referred to as capital costs and are not considered in this analysis. "A capital expenditure is a commitment of resources that is expected to provide benefits over a reasonably long period of time, at least two or more years."[5]

Table 2. Means and standard deviations for dependent variables

Dependent Variables	1980			1985			1990			1994		
	Mean	SD	N	Mean	SD	N	Mean	SD	N	Mean	SD	N
Efficiency outcomes												
expenses per adjusted admit ($1994)	2681	1053	4559	3640	1405	4503	4509	1724	4315	4884	1844	3957
full-time-equivalents per adj. census	3.24	0.75	4559	3.85	0.99	4503	4.15	1.23	4315	4.53	1.61	3957
Community-service outcomes												
ER visits per adj. inpatient day	0.27	0.16	4559	0.32	0.18	4503	0.37	0.21	4315	0.48	0.25	3957
outpatient visits per adj. inpatient. day	0.12	0.05	4559	0.18	0.06	4503	0.28	0.09	4315	0.36	0.11	3957

For purposes of standardization, the total hospital expenses were divided by the adjusted admissions.[6] Adjusted admissions are an "aggregate figure reflecting the number of days of inpatient care, plus an estimate of the volume of outpatient services, expressed in units equivalent to an inpatient day in terms of level of effort."[7]

Hospital strategies. Hospitals can implement various strategies in order to reduce costs. Examples of cost-reducing strategies include discontinuing unprofitable services, reducing the average length of stay, cost-shifting within the hospital, location choice, and the substitution of lower-skilled hospital personnel.

Historically, for-profit hospitals have avoided 'high-cost/ low-demand' services, such as burn units and neo-natal intensive-care units.[8] Policy analysts fear that all types of hospitals will scale back or cut unprofitable services in an effort to reduce their expenses. Emergency-rooms are typically not profitable, as they serve a disproportionate number of the underinsured and uninsured. Albrecht, Slobodkin and Rydman point out that a number of emergency departments and trauma centers have closed in recent years for reasons of unprofitability.[9]

In an effort to reduce costs, hospitals are also reducing their lengths of stay.[10] Implementation of the Prospective Payment System created an incentive for hospitals to shorten their average lengths of stay in an effort to reduce their overall treatment costs. In fact, "average length of stay per discharge dropped from 9.5 days in August 1983 to 7.5 days in August 1984."[11] In the years following passage of the Prospective Payment System, hospitals began releasing Medicare patients sooner after treatment than they had prior to PPS. Researchers subsequently found that these brief hospital stays were too short: often the patient returned to the hospital sicker than before the initial treatment. Health-service researchers began to refer to this phenomenon with the term "quicker and sicker."[12]

This phenomenon is not limited to Medicare patients. Following implementation of PPS, other third-party payors—including insurance companies and health maintenance organizations (HMOs)— adopted the capitated payment structure of the Prospective Payment System. To control their costs, these third-party payors limited their patients to prescribed lengths of hospitalization following treatment. Hospitals were forced to meet the demands of these third-party payors to ensure their future business. Hence expressions like "the drive-by delivery" and "the drive-by mastectomy" have entered everyday conversation. A study of a cost-cutting effort by executives and employees at the San Gabriel Valley Medical Center in California found that reducing the average length of stay reduces hospital costs. The hospital was able to decrease its average Medicare length of stay by one day (18 percent) by diagnosing and treating the patients earlier. The orthopedics department shortened its length of stay from 7 to 4.5 days by means of pre-operation home-care visits. This reduction in the length of stay saved approximately $2,000 per case.[13] In summary, hospitals have adopted the strategy of reducing their average lengths of stay in response to cost-reduction pressures from Medicare and other third-party payors.

Another cost reduction strategy is the art of locating in affluent areas. Norton and Staiger report that for-profit hospitals seek to locate in affluent areas to ensure a lower demand for charitable care.[14] That is, patients with employer provided health insurance utilize less charitable care than patients with Medicaid insurance. In fact, other researchers have found that for-profit hospitals seek to avoid caring for Medicaid patients: "For example, hospitals average more than 10 percent Medicaid patient days in twelve of Florida's fifty-nine counties. There are no investor owned hospitals in any of those twelve counties."[15] In many states, hospitals receive substantially lower reimbursements for Medicaid patients than from other third-party payors. And "some hospitals may also exclude Medicaid patients because they detract from the image they want to project to privately insured patients."[16]

Finally, hospitals can reduce their expenses per adjusted admission by substituting lower skilled aides and technicians for more highly skilled personnel. For instance, many hospitals are substituting aides and licensed practical nurses (LPNs) for more expensive registered nurses (RNs). Recent research indicates that a higher ratio of LPNs to RNs may not be in the best interest of the patient. In their study of hospital characteristics and mortality rates, Hartz and colleagues found that "lower adjusted mortality rates were associated with hospitals with a greater percentage of nurses who were RNs."[17] Additional research is needed to assess the effect of this trend on patient care.

Conclusion. Implementation of the Prospective Payment System has forced both not-for-profit and for-profit hospitals to reduce their operating expenses by means of various cost-reduction strategies. Until recently, few studies had analyzed the relationship between hospital costs and hospital performance. Two recent studies, however, demonstrate the importance of this relationship.

First, Burstin and colleagues examined the relationship between hospital operating costs and hospital quality using medical records from 51 acute-care hospitals in New York State. They assigned hospitals to quartiles based on their financial characteristics: hospitals with the highest operating costs were in quartile 4, hospitals with the lowest operating costs in quartile 1. They assessed hospital quality as the "percentage of adverse events due to negligence as evaluated by medical record review."[18] The researchers found a strong relationship between hospital costs and the risk of negligent injury. In fact, "patients admitted to hospitals with the lowest inpatient operating costs (quartile one) per hospital discharge were at greater risk of negligent injury. Moreover, hospitals under financial stress may spend less on patient care and may be more prone to injure patients through negligence."[19]

Second, in another study, Hartz and colleagues examined the relationship between hospital cost and hospital quality, using hospital mortality rates as a proxy for hospital quality. These results "suggest that greater financial stability may be associated with an improved quality of care."[20] In other words, Hartz and his colleagues found a relationship between a hospital's financial stability and lower mortality rate. Both of the above studies suggest that there is a relationship between a hospital's financial status and patient care.

As for-profit and not-for-profit hospitals continue to adopt similar cost-reduction strategies, the difference between the for-profit and not-for-profit hospital expenses per adjusted admission can be expected to narrow. Therefore, it is expected that hospital type will be less significant over time in explaining variations in hospital expenses per adjusted hospital admission.

Number of Full-Time-Equivalent Employees per Adjusted Census

Definition. The *number of full-time-equivalent employees per adjusted census* is also widely accepted as a proxy for hospital efficiency.[21] Hospital personnel are defined by the American Hospital Association as "full-time equivalents (FTEs), which are calculated by

adding the number of full-time personnel to one-half the number
of part-time personnel, excluding medical and dental residents
and interns and other trainees."[22] In order to standardize this figure, the ratio of FTEs to the adjusted census was used. The adjusted
census is the average number of patients (inpatients plus an equivalent figure for outpatients) receiving care during a given twelve-
month reporting period.[23]

Hospitals spend approximately 80 percent of their costs on
labor.[24] Employee labor, however, is one of the easiest components
for a hospital to control. Unlike capital expenditures, which are
fixed for long periods of time, many personnel-related decisions
are under managerial discretion and can be reduced in the short
run.[25] Hospitals can use various strategies to reduce the number of
their full-time-equivalent employees.

Hospital strategies. Barret explains that hospitals can realize
more cost savings by eliminating staff positions than by any other
mechanism.[26] "While a typical general hospital can switch from
thermal to flannel blankets in the nursery (saving $7,000 annu-
ally) and use natural rather than bleached paper towels (total savings $13,000), the biggest cuts in expenses come from eliminating
staff positions."[27] Researchers indicate that the cost-conscious
health-care environment has forced both for-profit and not-for-
profit hospitals to scrutinize their labor utilization. Conventional
wisdom once held that the strategy of staff reduction was limited
to for-profit hospitals. However many researchers find that not-
for-profit hospitals are also adopting such strategies.[28] It is difficult for hospitals to earn profits when they have high ratios of
FTEs per bed as labor is one of the most expensive components
of a hospital's operating budget. Therefore, researchers hypothesized that for-profit hospitals would have lower ratios of
FTEs than their not-for-profit counterparts. That is, the profit concerns of for-profit administrators would prompt them to limit
staff size.

In a 1985 study of Florida acute-care general hospitals, Sorrentino found that "for-profit hospital man-hours per patient day
were significantly lower than non-profit and government hospitals. . . . This indicates cost-cutting behavior on the part of a majority of for-profit hospitals. This method of limiting expenditures by
decreasing labor costs associated with certain services is consistent
with profit-maximization."[29] Recent data on acute-care hospitals,

mostly from Florida, suggest that the pattern of higher profits and lower staffing ratios at for-profit hospitals persist.[30]

Until recently, personnel-reduction strategies did not affect the physician staff. In recent years, however, the trend in staff reductions has extended to the medical staff. An outplacement firm in New York City predicts that, by the year 2000, 10 percent of the physicians in the New York City area may lose their jobs. According to the firm's projections, "doctors who are most vulnerable work in administration or in specialties such as cardiology, neurology, radiology, ophthalmology, anesthesiology, and urology. The more secure doctors work in primary care, family practice, and geriatrics."[31] The report also predicts that physicians who bring in more patients with shorter lengths of stays will be less likely to lose their positions than physicians who bring in fewer patients with longer lengths of stay.

Some researchers have found that administrative costs (e.g., the number of employees involved in administration) in American hospitals have increased over the past twenty years while the overall number of hospital patients has declined. Moreover, hospitals appear to be hiring administrative personnel at higher rates than patient-care personnel. According to Woolhandler and Himmelstein, "on an average day in 1968, U.S. hospitals employed 435,100 managers and clerks to assist in the care of 1,378,000 inpatients. By 1990, the average daily number of patients had fallen to 853,000; the number of administrators and clerks had risen to 1,221,600."[32][33]

In a more detailed analysis, Anderson and colleagues found that, from 1982 to 1994, the number of nonclinical hospital personnel in California increased more than twice as fast as the number of clinical personnel.[34] In another study, Shulkin and his colleagues found that the increasingly stringent regulation and cost-consciousness in the health-care environment has forced hospitals to hire administrative personnel at a faster rate than medical personnel.[35] Concern is growing that hospitals are willing to increase their administrative FTEs while reducing their medical FTEs—in other words, that they are pursuing efficiency rather than quality.

Conclusion. Traditionally, for-profit hospitals have been susceptible to more vigorous scrutiny by return-conscious boards than their not-for-profit counterparts. Research indicates, however, that the changing health-care environment has forced not-for-profit hospitals to behave like their for-profit counterparts.[36] Such trends suggest that both hospital types will use staff reduction as a means of cutting costs. Therefore, the impact of hospital type on the number of a hospital's FTEs per census can be expected to have declined from 1980 to 1994.

Community-Service Outcomes

Much of the health care literature suggests that when hospitals concentrate on efficiency they do so at the expense of community care. Some medical sociologists and health-services researchers worry that not-for-profit hospitals will abandon their community-service missions as they pursue cost-reducing strategies.[37] In particular, these researchers worry that hospitals will cut back on emergency services and outpatient services utilized disproportionately by the underinsured and uninsured.[38] Many of these emergency and outpatient services are unprofitable, and they are therefore defined by hospitals as community service. Research confirms that not-for-profit hospitals are more likely to provide services that are not moneymakers and that may in fact lose money. For instance, a recent report shows that "of the 4,376 AIDS care units in the nation, 81.6 percent are operated by not-for-profit hospitals compared with 8.2 percent by for-profit hospitals. And of the 881 trauma units nationwide, not-for-profit hospitals operate 91 percent, for-profits just 6.7 percent."[39] Recently, concern has been raised that many not-for-profit hospitals have begun to discontinue these types of services in an effort to reduce their expenses per adjusted admission.[40]

Two of the most common proxies for a hospital's provision of community service are emergency-room visits and outpatient visits.

Emergency-room Visits per Adjusted Inpatient Day

Definition. Many commentators see the emergency-room as the cornerstone of a hospital's provision of community care: "Emergency departments serve as the 7-Eleven of the medical world for a wide range of customers. They are the one-stop shopping sites for those who do not know where else to go. Emergency departments are open 24 hours a day, seven days a week, every day of the year. They are staffed by highly specialized teams who are used to assessing and dealing with every type of medical condition complicated by related social problems (such as alcohol, drugs, physical abuse and violence) under tight time constraints and with limited resources."[41] These demands make emergency departments expensive for hospitals to operate.[42]

Some studies use the mere absence or presence of an emergency department as an indicator of community service.[43] The present study examines the extent of emergency room services that hospitals provide. In order to standardize emergency-room utilization, the number of emergency-room visits were divided by adjusted inpatient days. Standardizing the number of emergency-room visits per adjusted inpatient day, makes it possible to compare the volume of emergency-room visits across hospital types over time.

Hospital strategies. Emergency departments must be staffed 24 hours a day, even when they are not busy; they must be at the technological cutting edge and they have high fixed costs.[44][45] Therefore, compared to other hospital departments, emergency departments are rarely successful profit centers. As Albrecht and his colleagues point out, "emergency departments are a risk center where ethical issues are raised and lawsuits are likely to originate."[46]

In the past few years, hospitals have seen an increase in patient demand for emergency-room services. In fact, the General Accounting Office reported that there were 99.6 million visits to emergency departments in 1990, an increase of 19 percent over 1985.[47] Nonurgent complaints accounted for a sizable portion of this increase in emergency-room utilization.[48] A disproportionate number of the people who use emergency-room for nonurgent care are uninsured and underinsured. Many of these patients use the emergency-room as their primary source of medical care.[49] In fact, "[t]he use of emergency departments for primary care has become so routine that some patients, particularly indigent ones, name their emergency-department physician when asked about their primary care-giver."[50] Of all health care for children with Medicaid insurance or no regular source of care, 28 percent occurs in the emergency-room.[51] On the other hand, "approximately 17 percent of all health care use for children with private health insurance and no regular source of care occurs in the emergency-room."[52] More than half of the 89.8 million emergency-department visits made in 1992 were for nonurgent care.[53] However, the primary care provided in the emergency room "lacks any element of continuity, is held to uncertain standards, and is frequently provided with marked lack of enthusiasm."[54] The overutilization of the emergency-room for nonurgent care, at a high cost to the public, prompted President Clinton to highlight the health-care savings that would be realized by reducing emergency-department utilization in his proposal for health-care reform.[55]

In addition to the demand for nonurgent care, emergency departments are expensive to operate because a high proportion of their patients are uninsured accident and trauma victims. These patients frequently require extensive and costly inpatient services, and hospitals are often unable to collect payment for their services.[56] Stern and colleagues, found that "patients admitted via the emergency department use far more resources than patients in the same diagnosis related group (DRG) admitted by other means."[57] These patients present special challenges in diagnosis, treatment or post-hospitalization placement.[58] Therefore, research indicates that hospitals with a high proportion of emergency admissions are likely to have high expenses per adjusted admission.[59]

Conclusion. Researchers emphasize that hospital efficiency and community care are inversely related. Many assert that hospital efficiency comes at the price of community. For instance, Kane argues that a hospital's positive financial performance, especially its ability to accumulate capital, exacts a price from the poor.[60] In a recent New York Times opinion piece, Brier discusses New York City's decision to lease its public hospitals to private health-care companies, thus relieving New York City of the financial burden of hospital management. She argues, however, that public hospitals in New York City care for people suffering from homelessness and drug and alcohol abuse who are generally unwelcome at other types of hospitals. Therefore, she warns, "selling or leasing city hospitals to companies whose primary concern is the bottom line will make it more difficult for these people to receive adequate care."[61]

Researchers disagree on the actual cost burden generated by the utilization of emergency departments for nonurgent care. Tyrance, Himmelstein and Woolhandler conclude that "emergency department use accounts for a small share of U.S. medical care costs, and cost shifting to the insured to cover free emergency department care for the uninsured is modest. Constraining emergency department use cannot generate substantial cost savings but may penalize minorities and the poor, who receive much of their outpatient care in emergency departments."[62] By contrast, a recent study by Ohio State University Hospital Researchers estimates that "$437 million in annual savings could be realized in Ohio alone if non-urgent emergency department visits were redirected to primary care physician's offices."[63] Whether hospitals cut emergency room services remains an empirical question. There is common ground, however, on two points. First, community residents see the emergency-room as one of the benefits that hospitals provide to their communities. Second, hospital administrators agree that emergency departments are expensive to operate and generally unprofitable, and that a large portion of this expense is attributable to care of the uninsured and underinsured.

Outpatient Visits as a Proportion of Adjusted Inpatient Days

Definition. A hospital's volume of outpatient visits is an appropriate proxy for community service, because it is a measure of the hospital's accessibility to the public. Outpatient services include clinics, crisis intervention, services to AIDS patients, medical tests and different types of screenings. Many of these services are disproportionately used by the underinsured and uninsured. Furthermore, Shortell reports that multi-hospital systems find many of these outpatient services unprofitable.[64] To compare the volume of outpatient care across hospitals, outpatient utilization was standardized by dividing the number of outpatient visits by adjusted inpatient days.

Hospital strategies. Patients who depend on hospital outpatient care experience lack of continuity with a primary caregiver, because residents generally rotate out of outpatient departments after a few months. Thus these individuals become the institution's patient's rather than a physician's patient. Ironically, these poorer patients need more continuity than their middle class-counterparts and receive less.[65] Poor minorities are more likely than other groups to utilize hospital outpatient departments on regular basis. "In 1989, 20 percent of blacks, compared to 12 percent of whites, reported in an annual federal health survey that their last contact with a physician had been at a hospital outpatient department. The gap between rich and poor was similar: 18 percent of survey respondents from families with incomes lower than $14,000 reported a hospital department as their last physician contact, compared to 11 percent of people with incomes higher than $50,000."[66] An outpatient department's volume is a good proxy for a hospital's provision of community service because hospital outpatient departments treat a disproportionate number of uninsured and underinsured patients.

Although there are problems inherent in the utilization of hospital outpatient departments for primary care, a recent study indicates that hospital outpatient clinics may offer more clinically effective and cost-effective care for some conditions than the hospital emergency-room. Moore and colleagues compared the morbidity and costs of treatment of two groups of patients with similar demographic and socioeconomic factors. These patients received asthma treatment at an inner city hospital, either in the emergency-room or at the allergy clinic. The study results indicate that treatment in the "allergy-immunology clinic is associated with better control of the disease than in the emergency-room. This suggests that early referral to the allergy-immunology clinic is important because it leads to reduced severity of asthma and decreased utilization of emergency-room services."[67]

A hospital's outpatient department is a costly mechanism for rendering patient care, and some fear that hospitals will abandon their provision of outpatient services. According to Goldsmith, Rush Presbyterian-St. Lukes Hospital and Medical Center in Chicago, adopted a sophisticated new organizational structure encompassing both horizontal and vertical integration, and now offers few outpatient services. The administrator who led the reorganization, "closed the hospital's outpatient department, which he considered to be an obsolete and excessively costly method of rendering care."[68] No alternate source of care was provided for the underinsured and uninsured.

Conclusion. Recently, Duffy and Farley analyzed prevailing financial incentives and organizational structures and their effect on the provision of hospital services. They found hospitals to be more efficient than in the 1970s; they also find that hospitals care for sicker and older patients in need of costly services. Duffy and Farley observe that the "continued squeezing to promote efficiency may begin to have unforeseen effects on the care of inpatients; ultimately, clinical effectiveness could be compromised."[69]

As hospitals are increasingly evaluated using efficiency indicators, we expect that this will come at a cost to the community. In other words, in their quest for efficiency, hospitals will bypass serving their communities. Therefore, we can expect that the difference between not-for-profit and for-profit hospitals' outpatient visits as a proportion of adjusted inpatient days will be greater in 1980 than in 1994.

SUMMARY

In previous studies, researchers have not simultaneously analyzed efficiency or community-service outcomes. Consequently, we know little about the relationship between hospital costs and community care. The research addresses this gap by analyzing both types of outcomes. This chapter presents a detailed description of the data and the four dependent variables used in the analysis. Each variable is defined and the strategies that hospitals use that affect these outcomes are analyzed. Many policy analysts fear that hospitals will abandon their community service missions in an effort to become more efficient. *Table 3* presents the correlations for the dependent variables used in the study. In the next chapter

Table 3. Correlations for dependent variables

Variable	expenses per adjusted admission	full-time equivalents per adjusted daily census	ER visits per adjusted inpatient day	outpatients visits per adjusted inpatient day
1980				
expenses per adjusted admission	1.000			
full-time equivalents per adjusted daily census	0.337 **	1.000		

Table 3. (Continued)

Variable	expenses per adjusted admission	full-time equivalents per adjusted daily census	ER visits per adjusted inpatient day	outpatients visits per adjusted inpatient day
ER visits per adjusted inpatient day	−0.038 **	0.289 **	1.000	
outpatient visits per adjusted inpatient day	0.007	0.071 **	0.352 **	1.000
1985				
expenses per adjusted admission	1.000			
full-time equivalents per adjusted daily census	0.150 **	1.000		
ER visits per adjusted inpatient day	−0.163 **	0.364 **	1.000	
outpatient visits per adjusted inpatient day	−0.160 **	0.067 **	0.310 **	1.000
1990				
expenses per adjusted admission	1.000			
full-time equivalents per adjusted daily census	0.150 **	1.000		
ER visits per adjusted inpatient day	−0.186 **	0.459 **	1.000	

Table 3. (Continued)

Variable	expenses per adjusted admission	full-time equivalents per adjusted daily census	ER visits per adjusted inpatient day	outpatients visits per adjusted inpatient day
outpatient visits per adjusted inpatient day 1994	−0.396 **	0.005	0.320 **	1.000
expenses per adjusted admission	1.000			
full-time equivalents per adjusted daily census	0.115 **	1.000		
ER visits per adjusted inpatient day	−0.158 **	0.485 **	1.000	
outpatient visits per adjusted inpatient day	−0.466 **	−0.030 **	0.211 **	1.000

**Correlation is significant at the 0.01 level (2-tailed)
*Correlation is significant at the 0.05 level (2-tailed)

organizational and environmental factors (independent variables) controlled for in the analysis are discussed.

NOTES

1. American Hospital Association, *1992 AHA Guide* (Chicago: American Hospital Association, 1992).

2. Complete AHA data sets (including hospitals with and without extrapolated data) were used for the creation of the Herfindahl Index, so

that the most accurate picture of the local hospital markets could be obtained (see page 84 for an explanation of the Herfindahl Index).

3. See R. E. Herzlinger, and W. S. Krasker, "Who Profits from Non-profits?" *Harvard Business Review* (1987): 93–105.

4. B. Arrington, and C. C. Haddock, "Who Really Profits from Not-For-Profits?" *Health Services Research* 25 (1990): 291–304.

5. W. O. Cleverly, *Essentials of Health Care Finance* (Gaithersburg, Maryland: Aspen Publishers, 1992), 365.

6. By standardizing the expenses by adjusted admission, expenses for hospitals with differences in their admission numbers can be compared (e.g., hospitals with 10,000 and 100,000 admissions).

7. American Hospital Association. *1994 AHA Guide* (Chicago: American Hospital Association, 1994), xxiv.

8. J. Greene, "A delicate balancing act," *Modern Healthcare* 25 (1995): 34–40; S. H. Altman, and D. Shactman. "Why should we worry about hospitals' high administrative costs?" *The New England Journal of Medicine.* 336 (1997): 798–99.

9. G. L. Albrecht, D. Slobodkin, , and R. J. Rydman. "The Role of Emergency Departments in American Health Care," In Research in the Sociology of Health Care, ed. J. J. Kronenfeld, (Greenwich, CT: JAI Press, 1996), 289–318.

10. K. Lumsdon, "Ready for Cost Cutting? One Hospital Mobilizes its Resources," *Hospital & Health Networks.* 68 (1994): 62.

11. Rosemary Stevens, *In Sickness and In Wealth: American Hospitals in the Twentieth Century* (New York: Basic Books, 1989), 326.

12. Senate Special Committee on Aging, *Quality of Care under Medicare's Prospective Payment System, Volume 1* (Washington DC: Government Printing Office, 1985); S. H. Altman, and D. A. Young "A Decade of Medicare's Prospective Payment System—Success or Failure?" *Journal of American Health Policy.* March/April (1993): 11–19.

13. K. Lumsdon, "Ready for Cost Cutting?"

14. E. C. Norton, and D. O. Staiger, "How Hospitals Ownership Affects Access to Care for the Uninsured," *Rand Journal of Economics* 25 (1994): 171–85.

15. C. G. Homer, D. D. Bradham, and M. Rushefsky, "To the Editor, Investor-Owned and Not-For-Profit Hospitals: Beyond the Cost and Revenue Debate," *Health Affairs* (1984): 134.

16. Ibid.

17. A. J. Hartz, H. Krakauer, E. M. Kuhn, M. Young, S. J. Jacobsen, G. Greer, L. Muenz, M. Katzoff, R. C. Bailey, and A. A. Rimm, "Hospital Char-

acteristics and Mortality Rates," *The New England Journal of Medicine.* 321 (1989): 1720–1725.

18. "Adverse events are injuries caused by medical management, as opposed to underlying disease process. Adverse events can then be further classified as negligent or not negligent. The negligence determination is based on the reviewer's assessment of compliance with the standards expected of the reasonable medical practitioner." See H. R. Burstin, S. R. Lipsitz, S. Udvarhelyi, and T. A. Brennan, "The Effect of Hospital Financial Characteristics on Quality of Care," *Journal of the American Medical Association* 270 (1993): 847.

19. Ibid., 848.

20. Hartz et al., "Hospital Characteristics and Mortality Rates," 1724.

21. Arrington, and Haddock, "Who Really Profits from Not-For-Profits?"

22. American Hospital Association, *1994 AHA Guide,* xxiv).

23. Ibid., xxiii.

24. G. F. Anderson, and L. T. Kohn, "Hospital Employment Trends in California, 1982–1994," *Health Affairs* 15 (1996): 152–158.

25. Ibid.

26. M. W. Barrett, "Downsizing: Doing it Rationally," *Nursing Management* 26 (1995): 24–29.

27. Ibid., 24.

28. Paul Starr, *The Social Transformation of American Medicine* (New York: Basic Books, 1982); Rosemary Stevens, *In Sickness and In Wealth;* M. L. Fennel, and J. A. Alexander, "Perspectives on Organizational Change in the US Medical Sector," *Annual Review of Sociology* 19 (1993): 89–112.

29. E. A. Sorrentino, "Hospital Mission and Cost Differences," *Hospital Topics* 67 (1989): 24.

30. S. Woolhandler, and D. U. Himmelstein. "Costs of care and administration at for-profit and other hospitals in the United States," *The New England Journal of Medicine* 336 (1997): 769–74.

31. Hospitals & Health Networks, "Human Resources," *Hospitals & Health Networks,* October 20 (1996):11.

32. S. Woolhandler, D. U. Himmelstein, and J. P. Lewontin, "Administrative Costs in U.S. Hospitals," *The New England Journal of Medicine* 329 (1993): 401.

33. Woolhandler and Himmelstein (1991, 1993, 1997) continually critique administrative costs in U.S. hospitals. They often suggest that the Canadian system as an alternative model. In a letter to the *New England Journal of Medicine,* U.S. Representative Bill Archer of Texas argues that

"the Canadian model that Woolhandler and Himmelstein advocate for this country is not so enticing. Rates of growth in per capita expenses in Canada and the United States during the past decade are comparable, despite the use of price and budget controls in Canada. Furthermore, examples abound of long queues and lack of access to sophisticated medical care in Canada. Before we rush to replicate the Canadian system, we need to examine and understand its problems." See B. Archer, "To the Editor," *The New England Journal of Medicine* 325 (1991): 1316.

34.   Anderson, and Kohn, "Hospital Employment Trends in California."

35.   D. J. Shulkin, A. L. Hillman, and W. M. Cooper, "Reasons for Increasing Administrative Costs in Hospitals," *Annals of Internal Medicine* 119 (1993): 74–78.

36.   See Paul Starr, *The Social Transformation of American Medicine;* Rosemary Stevens, *In Sickness and In Wealth;* Fennel, and Alexander, "Perspectives on Organizational Change."

37.   Rosemary Stevens, *In Sickness and In Wealth;* Fennel, and Alexander, "Perspectives on Organizational Change."

38.   "Despite public and private insurance programs about one-third of U.S. citizens are without health insurance or had difficulty getting or paying for medical care at some time last year. . . . 40 million adults were uninsured in 1995 or at some time in the prior year. . . . Excluding the elderly and members of the military and their families—who are covered by the federal government—the majority of the uninsured are full-time workers (about 41 percent)." See D. Kendall, *Social Problems in a Diverse Society* (London: Allyn and Bacon, 1998), 243.

39.   F. Cerne, "Street Wise: Analysts upbeat about providers' response to volatile market," *Hospitals & Health Networks* (1995): 42.

40.   M. A. Morrisey, G. J. Wedig, and M. Hassan, "Do Nonprofit Hospital Pay Their Way?" *Health Affairs* 15 (1996): 132–144.

41.   G. L. Albrecht, D. Slobodkin, and R. J. Rydman, "The Role of Emergency Departments in American Health Care," In *Research in the Sociology of Health Care*, ed. J. J. Kronenfeld, (Greenwich, CT: JAI Press, 1996), 290.

42.   Ibid.

43.   S. M. Shortell, E. M. Morrison, S. L. Hughes, B. Friedman, J. Coverdill, and L. Berg. "The Effects of Hospital Ownership on Nontraditional Services," *Health Affairs* Winter (1986): 97–111.

44.   Albrecht, et. al., "The Role of Emergency Departments;" P. H. Tyrance, D. U. Himmelstein, and S. Woolhandler, "US Emergency Department Costs: No Emergency," *American Journal of Public Health* 86 (1996): 1527–1531.

45.   "A resource is a fixed cost if the amount consumed does not vary with volume. For example, if a bypass pump can handle up to 250 patients per year, the high volume center might need one, whereas the low-volume centers would need one each. Total costs would be higher for two centers than for one, since two pumps are used instead of one. This assumes that extra costs of centralization such as increased travel do not more than off-set the cost of the additional pump." See S. A. Finkler, "The Distinction Between Cost and Charges," *Annals of Internal Medicine* 96 (1982): 103.

46.   Albrecht, et. al., "The Role of Emergency Departments," 291.

47.   General Accounting Office, "Report to the chairman, Subcommittee on Health for Families and the Uninsured, Committee on Finance, U.S. Senate: emergency departments unevenly affected by growth and change in patient use," Publication no. GAO/HRD-93-4, (Washington D.C.: Government Printing Office, 1993); R.M. Williams, "The Costs of Visits to Emergency Departments," *TheNew England Journal of Medicine* 334 (1996): 642–646.

48.   Tyrance, et. al., "US Emergency Department Costs."

49.   Albrecht, et. al., "The Role of Emergency Departments."

50.   P. McNamara, R. Witte, and A. Koning, "Patchwork Access: Primary Care in EDs on the rise," *Hospitals* (1993): 45.

51.   S. T. Orr, E. Charney, J. Strauss, and B. Bloom, "Emergency Room Use by Low Income Children with a Regular Source of Health Care," *Medical Care* 29 (1991): 283–286.

52.   Ibid., 285.

53.   D. W. Baker, C. Stevens, and R. H. Brook, "Determinants of Emergency Department Use by Ambulatory Patients at an Urban Public Hospital," *Annals of Emergency Medicine* 25 (1995): 311–316.

54.   Albrecht, et. al., "The Role of Emergency Departments," 296; also see Baker et al., "Determinants of Emergency Department Use."

55.   Tyrance, et. al., "US Emergency Department Costs."

56.   Committee on Implications of For-Profit Enterprise in Health Care, "Access to Care," In *For-Profit Enterprise in Health Care* ed. B. H. Gray, Washington, DC: National Academy Press, 1986); Arrington and Haddock, Who Profits from Nonprofits."

57.   R. S. Stern, J. S. Weissman, and A. M. Epstein, "The Emergency Department as a Pathway to Admission for Poor and High-Cost Patients," *Journal of the American Medical Association* 266 (1991): 2238.

58.   Ibid.

59.   Some recent research indicates that diverting nonurgent cases from the emergency room to private physicians would not result in large cost

savings. See R. M. Williams, "The Costs of Visits to Emergency Departments." *The New England Journal of Medicine* 334 (1996): 642–646. In fact, one study found that the cost differences between treatment of a patient in an emergency department and treating the same patient in a nonemergency department is only approximately $65 (Baker and Baker 1994). Moreover, Tyrance, Himmelstein and Woolhandler argue that, since emergency department already have high fixed costs, their costs to accommodate nonemergency visits are incidental. Therefore, these researchers argue that though the $200 charge for treatment of a migraine headache in an emergency department may seem wasteful, the costs to society as a whole of shifting this care to a primary-care physician may be higher. See Tyrance, et. al., "US Emergency Department Costs." See also A. L. Kellerman, "Nonurgent Emergency Department Visits: Meeting an Unmet Need," *Journal of the American Medical Association* 271 (1994): 1953–1954.

60.   Nancy Kane, "Report on the Financial Resources of Major Hospitals in Boston." (Department of Health and Hospitals:Boston, 1993).

61.   P. Brier, "At Risk: Health Care for the Poor," *New York Times* (January 18, 1997):21.

62.   Tyrance, et. al., "US Emergency Department Costs."

63.   McNamara, Witte, and Koning, "Patchwork Access: Primary Care in Eds," 46.

64.   S. M. Shortell, "The Evolution of Hospital Systems: Unfulfilled Promises and Self-Fulfilling Prophesies," *Medical Care Review* 45 (1988): 177–213.

65.   L. K. Abraham, *Mama Might Be Better Off Dead: The Failure of Health Care in America* (Chicago: The University of Chicago Press, 1993).

66.   Ibid.; E. J. Goodwin, et al. "Access to Health Care: Medicare and the Poor Elderly," In *Poverty and Health in the United States*, ed. M. I. Krasner (New York: United Hospital Fund, 1989).

67.   C. M. Moore, I. Ahmed, R. Mouallem, W. May, M. Ehlayel, and R. U. Sorensen. "Care of Asthma: Allergy Clinic Versus Emergency Room" *Annals of Allergy, Asthma and Immunology* 78 (1997): 379.

68.   Jeff C. Goldsmith, *Can Hospital's Survive?* (Homewood, Illinois: Dow Jones-Irwin,1981),151.

69.   Sarah Q. Duffy, and Dean E. Farley, "Patterns of Decline among Inpatient Procedures," *Public Health Reports* 11 (1995): 680.

CHAPTER 4

Hospitals' Organizational Characteristics and Environments

In order to examine claims of a narrowing distinction between hospital types, it is important to control for factors that could confound the analysis. These factors were divided into two categories: internal organizational factors and environmental characteristics. This chapter examines each of these factors.

HOSPITAL INTERNAL ORGANIZATIONAL CHARACTERISTICS

Many studies have analyzed internal factors to determine whether the distinction between hospital types is narrowing.[1] The underlying logic is that these internal factors influence the outcomes (dependent variables) described in Chapter 3; thus for-profit and not-for-profit hospitals that share the same internal characteristics have similar outcomes.

Controlling for internal factors that previous research has found to be significant enables the author to evaluate the efficiency and community-service outcomes used to asses claims of a declining distinction between hospital types. These internal factors include ownership type, hospital-system affiliation, size, teaching status, case mix, the ratio of technology services, average length of stay, and the ratio of full-time licensed practical nurses (LPNs) to full-time registered nurses (RNs). In the following section these factors are defined and discuss the importance of controlling for each of these variables is discussed. *Table 4,* presents the means and standard deviations for these variables for each year of the study.

Type of Ownership

A historical and analytical description of the four categories of hospital ownership used in this analysis—for-profit, private not-for-profit, religious not-for-profit and government not-for-profit—appears in Chapter 3. The government not-for-profit category of hospital ownership is used as the reference category in the multiple regression analysis.

Hospital-System Affiliation

Since 1980, the American Hospital Association (AHA) Annual Survey has identified those hospitals that belong to multi-hospitals systems. The AHA defines a multi-hospital health-care system as "two or more hospitals owned, leased, sponsored or contract managed by a central organization."[2] This research controls for the absence or presence of a multi-hospital system affiliation. Some researchers posit that organizational affiliation offers a stronger explanation than organizational type (i.e., for-profit or not-for-profit) for variations in organizational performance.[3]

In a study of the behavior of home health agencies, for example, Estes and Swan (1994) find that not-for-profit system-affiliated home health agencies behave more like for-profit home health agencies than like independent not-for-profit home health agencies.[4] This finding is consistent with neo-institutional theory. These theorists recognize that the organizational affiliations, in addition to organizational type, offer explanatory power for variation in organizational outcomes.

System affiliation provides hospitals with many benefits. For example, Becker and Sloan refer to the distinction between chain and independent hospitals as a key organizational characteristic: "The chains often assert that their size enables them to purchase non-labor inputs for less. Moreover, they offer better opportunities for career advancement and therefore can hire more capable employees for a given level of pay."[5] Furthermore, some evidence suggests that hospitals in systems are less costly to operate than

Table 4. Means and standard deviations for internal independent variables

Independent Variables	1980			1985			1990			1994		
	Mean	SD	N	Mean	SD	N	Mean	SD	N	Mean	SD	N
hospital ownership type (government not-for-profit hospitals are the reference category)												
government not-for-profit hospital	0.287	0.452	4559	0.262	0.440	4503	0.257	0.437	4315	0.254	0.435	3957
for-profit hospital	0.107	0.310	4559	0.123	0.329	4503	0.126	0.332	4315	0.113	0.317	3957
private not-for-profit hospital	0.468	0.499	4559	0.479	0.500	4503	0.486	0.500	4315	0.507	0.500	3957
religious not-for-profit hospital	0.138	0.345	4559	0.136	0.343	4503	0.132	0.338	4315	0.126	0.332	3957
system affiliation												

Table 4. (Continued)

Independent Variables	1980			1985			1990			1994		
	Mean	SD	N	Mean	SD	N	Mean	SD	N	Mean	SD	N
member of a hospital system	0.250	0.433	4559	0.410	0.492	4503	0.469	0.499	4315	0.531	0.499	3957
hospital size (hospitals with fewer than 100 beds are the reference category)												
fewer than 100 beds	0.429	0.495	4559	0.413	0.492	4503	0.413	0.493	4315	0.411	0.492	3957
100 to 249 beds	0.320	0.467	4559	0.329	0.470	4503	0.330	0.470	4315	0.341	0.474	3957
250 to 399 beds	0.142	0.349	4559	0.149	0.356	4503	0.153	0.360	4315	0.147	0.354	3957
400 or more beds	0.108	0.311	4559	0.109	0.311	4503	0.104	0.306	4315	0.101	0.301	3957
hospital teaching status												
member of Council of Teaching	0.050	0.218	4559	0.064	0.244	4503	0.056	0.229	4315	0.057	0.231	3957

Table 4. (Continued)

Independent Variables	1980			1985			1990			1994		
	Mean	SD	N	Mean	SD	N	Mean	SD	N	Mean	SD	N
Hospitals (COTH)												
medical-school affiliation	0.081	0.272	4559	0.094	0.292	4503	0.121	0.326	4315	0.134	0.340	3957
intern or residency program	0.050	0.218	4559	0.034	0.182	4503	0.030	0.170	4315	0.045	0.207	3957
hospital case-mix indicators												
proportion of operations that are inpatient operations	0.855	0.154	4559	0.666	0.158	4503	0.463	0.148	4315	0.384	0.148	3957
Medicaid inpatient days as a proportion of adjusted inpatient days	0.069	0.050	4559	0.085	0.075	4503	0.093	0.084	4315	0.107	0.099	3957

Table 4. (Continued)

Independent Variables	1980			1985			1990			1994		
	Mean	SD	N	Mean	SD	N	Mean	SD	N	Mean	SD	N
Medicare inpatient days as a proportion of adjusted inpatient days	0.386	0.116	4559	0.369	0.111	4503	0.343	0.114	4315	0.318	0.125	3957
other internal hospital characteristics												
ratio of full-time LPNs to full-time RNs	0.333	0.167	4559	0.270	0.154	4503	0.242	0.155	4315	0.206	0.148	3957
average length of stay using inpatient days	7.238	2.732	4559	6.838	3.815	4503	7.626	5.662	4315	7.237	7.428	3957
ratio of technology services	0.311	0.300	4559	0.331	0.263	4503	0.353	0.292	4315	0.413	0.304	3957

independent hospitals. Menke compared the cost structures of hospitals in multi-hospital systems and independently owned hospitals, and he found that hospitals with system affiliations are better equipped than independent hospitals to take advantage of economies of scale.[6] These findings are consistent with other studies of hospital performance in multi-hospital systems.[7]

Since 1980, the number of hospitals with system affiliations has increased (see *Table 5*). In fact, only 25 percent of all hospitals had system affiliations in 1980, compared with 53 percent of all hospitals in 1994—an increase of over 100 percent. Additionally, the percentage of hospitals with system affiliations has increased among all four

Table 5. Hospitals with system affiliations by type and year

Hospital Type	Number and percent of hospitals affiliated with a system							
	1980		1985		1990		1994	
	N	n (%)	N	n (%)	N	n (%)	N	n (%)
for-profit	490	332 (68%)	556	419 (75%)	544	432 (79%)	447	375 (84%)
private not-for-profit	2132	339 (16%)	2155	692 (32%)	2096	836 (40%)	2006	985 (49%)
religious not-for profit	630	254 (40%)	613	427 (70%)	568	462 (81%)	498	419 (84%)
government not-for-profit	1307	214 (16%)	1179	306 (26%)	1107	293 (26%)	1006	322 (32%)
Total	4559	1139 (25%)	4503	1844 (41%)	4315	2023 (47%)	3957	2101 (53%)

N: number of hospitals
n: number of hospitals that are affiliated with a system
%: percent of hospitals that are affiliated with a system

hospital types. When analyzing distinctions between hospital types, therefore, it is important to control for a hospital's system affiliation.

Hospital Size

Hospital size is controlled for in order to ensure that similarities in hospital outcomes are not a function of hospital size. Researchers use the number of beds, cribs and pediatric bassinets that a hospital maintains on a regular basis as a proxy for hospital size. [8] Health services researchers find that the average cost per bed rises as the size of the hospital (e.g., number of beds) increases. Their findings stand in stark contrast to research in other industries, which finds the average cost of production decreases as average size increases (i.e., economies of scale). Large hospitals, however, have not been able to exploit economies of scale, at least with regard to cost. This would occur because the largest hospitals are located in expensive urban areas; many of these urban hospitals are teaching hospitals and a high proportion of their patients are uninsured.[9]

Over the past fifteen years, the mean number of beds at for-profit hospitals has slightly increased; at government and private not-for-profit hospitals it has remained constant. Meanwhile, the mean number of beds at religious not-for-profit hospitals has minimally decreased (*see Table 6*).

In recent years, many researchers have found that not-for-profit hospitals have become increasingly cost-conscious. One strategy these hospitals use to reduce their costs and increase revenues is to reduce the number of beds and to use this space for more profitable endeavors. For example, some hospitals have converted such space into higher revenue producing private rooms and suites, restaurants and other retail establishments.[10] Thus research demonstrates the importance of controlling for hospital size when analyzing claims of a declining distinction between hospital types. This research uses four categories of hospital size; fewer than 100 beds, 100–249 beds, 250–399 beds and 400 or more beds. Hospitals with fewer than 100 beds is used as the reference category.

Teaching Status

The availability of training opportunities for medical students, residents, physicians and other medical professionals is controlled for

Table 6. Hospital size by hospital type, 1980–1994

Hospital Type	1980		1985		1990		1994	
	Mean*	SD	Mean*	SD	Mean*	SD	Mean*	SD
for-profit	132.95	89.42	131.15	89.96	145.81	95.21	152.95	100.70
private not-for-profit	201.11	175.20	207.65	182.00	204.51	175.80	200.81	176.50
religious not-for-profit	282.16	208.50	279.23	208.30	263.70	197.60	252.58	197.30
government not-for-profit	117.24	137.20	125.45	159.20	121.21	156.30	121.17	156.80

*The mean number of hospital beds.

in this analysis in order to ensure that similarities in organizational outcomes are not merely a function of a hospital's teaching status. Research has shown that hospital training programs are costly to provide.[11] In fact, a 1989 General Accounting Office study found that in 1985 "the average Medicare cost per discharge was 95 percent higher at a major teaching hospital than at a non-teaching hospital, and 39 percent higher than at a minor teaching hospital."[12] The higher costs of teaching hospitals are a result of both direct costs and indirect costs. Indirect costs are those costs resulting from increased diagnostic testing, an increase in the number of procedures performed, higher staffing ratios and increased record keeping. Alternately, direct costs include "salary and fringes for residents, interns, and teaching physicians, conference and classroom space, additional equipment, supplies, and allocated overhead on these items."[13] Teaching hospitals are costly endeavors for several other reasons.

Teaching hospitals treat a more costly mix of patients, maintain larger reserve margins, have larger staffs and offer more extensive treatment options.[14] For the most part, teaching hospitals are private not-for-profit and religious not-for-profit hospitals *(see Table 7)*. Traditionally, teaching hospitals provide a wider range of medical services than do nonteaching hospitals. These diverse services contribute to higher expenses per hospital admission. Teaching hospitals are also disproportionately located in major urban areas, and are often larger than their non-teaching counterparts. Teaching hospitals generally care for disproportionate numbers of the uninsured and patients with more serious conditions. These hospitals are typically not reimbursed the full cost of such care. Furthermore, the cost of attracting and retaining high-quality physicians also accounts for higher costs at teaching hospitals.[15] Finally, "besides providing patient care, teaching hospitals function as a clinical training site for new physicians. Many believe that the latest in medical technology must be made available in order to train young physicians and provide clinical research opportunities."[16]

Research that focuses on hospitals' teaching status usually differentiates three levels of teaching commitment. The level of a hospital's teaching commitment "has a substantial effect on case mix complexity and . . . this effect increases with the degree of commitment."[17] Therefore, this study treats the following three levels of hospital teaching status as independent variables: (1) whether

Table 7. COTH membership by hospital type, 1980–1994

Hospital Type	1980 N	1980 n (%)	1985 N	1985 n (%)	1990 N	1990 n (%)	1994 N	1994 n (%)
for-profit	490	0 (0%)	556	3 (1%)	544	2 (0%)	447	2 (0%)
private not-for-profit	2132	145 (7%)	2155	168 (8%)	2096	145 (7%)	2006	141 (7%)
religious not-for-profit	630	37 (6%)	613	54 (9%)	568	34 (6%)	498	30 (6%)
government not-for-profit	1307	47 (4%)	1179	62 (5%)	1107	59 (5%)	1006	51 (5%)
total	4559	229 (5%)	4503	287 (6%)	4315	240 (6%)	3957	224 (6%)

N: number of hospitals
n: number of hospitals that are members of COTH
%: percent of hospitals that are members of COTH

the hospital is a member of the council of teaching hospitals (COTH), (2) whether the hospital is affiliated with a medical school and (3) whether the hospital has an intern or residency program. Each variable is coded "1" if the hospital has the attribute and "0" if it does not.[18]

Council of Teaching Hospitals (COTH)

Membership in the Council of Teaching Hospitals of the Association of American Medical Colleges signifies the highest level of teaching commitment. In 1994 only 6 percent of all hospitals were COTH members, a percentage that has remained fairly constant over the past fifteen years (see *Table 7*). The majority of COTH members are private not-for-profit hospitals and religious not-for-profit hospitals. Compared with the other two types of teaching affiliations, COTH membership signifies the presence of extensive and costly services. Thorpe explains that COTH hospitals "have significantly higher ratios of skilled nursing and total nursing staff per bed than do other hospitals. Moreover, COTH hospitals employ a significantly higher ratio of skilled to licensed practical nurses than do non-teaching facilities."[19]

Medical-School Affiliation

Compared to membership in COTH, medical-school affiliation represents the second-highest commitment to medical training. In 1994, approximately 13 percent of hospitals had a medical-school affiliation (see *Table 8*). The proportion of such hospitals has slightly increased over the past 15 years. Most are religious not-for-profit hospitals and private not-for-profit hospitals.

Table 8. Medical-school affiliation by hospital type, 1980–1994

Hospital Type	1980		1985		1990		1994	
	N	n (%)	N	n (%)	N	n (%)	N	n (%)
for-profit	490	3 (1%)	556	4 (1%)	544	19 (3%)	447	17 (4%)
private not-for-profit	2132	196 (9%)	2155	243 (11%)	2096	300 (14%)	2006	335 (17%)
religious not-for profit	630	121 (19%)	613	130 (21%)	568	148 (26%)	498	126 (25%)
government not-for-profit	1307	47 (4%)	1179	45 (4%)	1107	53 (5%)	1006	51 (5%)
total	4559	367 (8%)	4503	422 (9%)	4315	520 (12%)	3957	529 (13%)

N: number of hospitals
n: number of hospitals that have medical school affiliations
%: percent of hospitals that have medical school affiliations

Intern or Residency program

The presence of an internship or residency program represents the lowest level of teaching commitment. This category includes hospitals approved to participate in residency training by the Accreditation Council for Graduate Medical Education as well as hospitals with internship and residency programs approved by the American Osteopathic Association. Approximately 4 percent of the hospitals had intern or residency programs in 1994 (see *Table 9*). The proportion of such hospitals has remained fairly constant over the past 15 years. Most are private not-for-profit and religious not-for-profit hospitals.

Table 9. Presence of an intern or residency program by hospital type, 1980–1994

Hospital Type	1980		1985		1990		1994	
	N	n (%)	N	n (%)	N	n (%)	N	n (%)
for-profit	490	12 (2%)	556	12 (2%)	544	26 (5%)	447	27 (6%)
private not-for-profit	2132	150 (7%)	2155	109 (5%)	2096	84 (4%)	2006	108 (5%)
religious not-for-profit	630	51 (8%)	613	21 (3%)	568	15 (3%)	498	31 (6%)
government not-for-profit	1307	16 (1%)	1179	12 (1%)	1107	4 (0%)	1006	12 (1%)
total	4559	229 (5%)	4503	154 (3%)	4315	129 (3%)	3957	178 (4%)

N: number of hospitals
n: number of hospitals that have intern or residency programs
%: percent of hospitals that have intern or residency programs

Hospital Case Mix

The hospital's case mix is controlled for in order to ensure that similarities in hospital outcomes are not a function of hospital case mix. The importance of controlling for hospital case mix has been well documented in the health-services literature: as Sloan and Becker point out, "it is widely recognized that hospital case mix is a major determinant of hospital costliness."[20] Therefore, this analysis controls for three internal determinants of a hospital's case mix: (1) the proportion of surgical operations that are inpatient surgeries, (2) Medicaid inpatient days as a proportion of adjusted inpatient days and (3) Medicare inpatient days as a proportion of adjusted inpatient days.

Proportion of Surgical Operations that are Inpatient Surgeries

The proportion of surgical operations that are inpatient surgeries is a proxy for the complexity of a hospital's case mix. Generally speaking, inpatient surgeries are more serious than outpatient surgeries, and hospitals with a high proportion of inpatient operations tend to see patients in need of complex services.[21] Therefore, a high level of inpatient surgery suggests a more intensive hospital environment. Conversely, hospitals that perform a limited number of inpatient operations see relatively minor cases.

Recent studies have examined the relationships among hospital surgical volume and patient mortality rates.[22] Hospitals and surgeons with a high volume of specific surgeries have lower mortality rates than hospitals with low surgical volumes. As Stevens observes, "it is not surprising, then, that hospitals seeking to qualify for Medicare reimbursement for cardiac transplantation now have to meet specified conditions. These include preexisting open-heart surgery programs that perform at least 250 procedures a year, at least twelve heart transplants (on persons of any age) in each of the past two years, and specified survival rates (seventy-three percent after one year and sixty-five percent after two years), together with other criteria."[23] Table 10 presents inpatient surgeries as a proportion of all surgeries.

Medicaid Inpatient Days as a Proportion of Adjusted Inpatient Days

Individuals are eligible for Medicaid benefits when their incomes are below the state-mandated poverty level. Compared with non-

Table 10. Proportion of surgical operations that are inpatient by hospital type, 1980–1994

Hospital Type	1980		1985		1990		1994	
	*Mean	SD	Mean	SD	Mean	SD	Mean	SD
for-profit	0.878	0.141	0.685	0.152	0.454	0.131	0.387	0.137
private not-for-profit	0.838	0.151	0.641	0.150	0.458	0.138	0.386	0.139
religious not-for-profit	0.856	0.118	0.662	0.131	0.478	0.128	0.406	0.122
government not-for-profit	0.873	0.172	0.706	0.179	0.467	0.181	0.368	0.178

* Mean inpatient surgery ratio

Medicaid recipients, Medicaid recipients are less likely to have a private physician. Researchers have found that patients without private doctors use $228 more a year in outpatient-department services and $375 a year more in overall medical services than patients with private doctors.[24] In some states, Medicaid recipients have difficulty finding a private physician. For instance William D. Pike, president of the Western New York Hospital Association, explains that New York Medicaid's low reimbursement rate for a physician visit, $7, effectively discourages physicians from participating in the Medicaid program. Hospital emergency departments thus treat a high volume of Medicaid patients who have nowhere else to go.[25] Pike adds that "may of these patients show up sicker than if they had had timely access to comprehensive primary care."[26] Therefore, Medicaid patients are more costly to treat than patients with other types of insurance.

Since Medicaid reimbursement rates are quite low in some states, hospitals may not be fully reimbursed. In a study comparing investor-owned and voluntary hospital systems, Cleverly found that many investor-owned hospital systems associate treatment of Medicaid patients with higher levels of bad debt and charity care; therefore it is more profitable for a hospital to avoid these patients.[27] Since Medicaid patients often present sicker than patients with other types of insurance, and hospitals generally do not receive full compensation for treating Medicaid patients, it is important to control for the proportion of Medicaid inpatient days as one proxy for a hospital's case mix. Table 11 presents Medicaid inpatient days as a proportion of adjusted inpatient days.

Medicare Inpatient Days as a Proportion of Adjusted Inpatient Days

Patients age 65 and older have more intensive health-care needs than their younger counterparts. According to a recent study of emergency-department utilization, patients age 65 and over utilize emergency-rooms less than their younger counterparts.[28] When such patients are admitted to the emergency-room, however, they use more hospital services than younger patients.[29] In fact, compared with patients under the age 65, the elderly are more likely to use ambulance transport, to be admitted to the hospital, to be admitted to an intensive care bed, and to receive care classified as a comprehensive emergency-department level

Table 11. Medicaid inpatient days as a proportion of adjusted inpatient days, by hospital type, 1980–1994

Hospital Type	1980		1985		1990		1994	
	*Mean	SD	Mean	SD	Mean	SD	Mean	SD
for-profit	0.07	0.06	0.07	0.06	0.08	0.07	0.10	0.08
private not-for-profit	0.07	0.05	0.08	0.07	0.09	0.08	0.11	0.10
religious not-for-profit	0.07	0.04	0.08	0.07	0.09	0.07	0.10	0.09
government not-for-profit	0.07	0.05	0.10	0.08	0.11	0.10	0.12	0.11

*Mean Medicaid inpatient ratio

of service.[30] Compared to younger adults, furthermore, adults 65 and over who are admitted to emergency departments use more laboratory and radiology tests.[31] Because of these differences between Medicare patients, and non-Medicare patients, it is necessary to control for the hospital's proportion of Medicare patients. Table 12 presents Medicare inpatient days as a proportion of adjusted inpatient days by hospital type.

Average Length of Stay

The hospital's average length of stay is controlled for in order to ensure that the differences in hospital outcomes are not attributable to the hospital's average length of stay. The average length of stay in short-term general hospitals in 1994 was approximately seven days.[32] Table 13 presents average length of stay by hospital type for each year of the study. Historically, government not-for-profit hospitals have had longer lengths of stay than hospitals that treat fewer uninsured and underinsured patients (see Chapter 2). Generally speaking, hospitals with longer lengths of stay tend to treat sicker patients.

Increased utilization of price controls in the health-care system has created incentives for hospitals to release their patients earlier. Many medical researchers debate the implications for patients' health and recovery of reducing the average length of stay.[33] Many of these researchers argue that patients who are recovering well are not put at risk of further complications by being released earlier. Others point out that patients experiencing prolonged stays are more likely to suffer complications, including adverse drug events.[34] In fact, Classen and colleagues found that adverse drug events were associated with an increased length of stay of approximately two days. By controlling for average length of stay, it is possible to control for the types of patients that hospitals treat.

**Ratio of Full-Time Licensed Practical Nurses
to Full-Time Registered Nurses**

In this analysis hospital's staffing arrangements are controlled for in order to ensure that variation in hospital outcomes are not a function of hospital labor practices. Therefore, controlling for a hospital's ratio of full-time licensed practical nurses (LPNs) to full-time

Table 12. Medicare inpatient days as a proportion of adjusted inpatient days, by hospital type

Hospital Type	1980		1985		1990		1994	
	*Mean	SD	Mean	SD	Mean	SD	Mean	SD
For-profit	0.40	0.12	0.37	0.11	0.37	0.11	0.37	0.12
Private not-for-profit	0.38	0.11	0.37	0.10	0.34	0.11	0.32	0.12
Religious not-for-profit	0.38	0.10	0.37	0.09	0.36	0.10	0.34	0.11
Government not-for-profit	0.39	0.13	0.36	0.13	0.32	0.13	0.28	0.14

*Mean Medicare inpatient ratio

Table 13. Average length of stay (ALOS) by hospital type

Hospital Type	1980		1985		1990		1994	
	*Mean	SD	Mean	SD	Mean	SD	Mean	SD
for-profit	6.67	1.91	5.85	1.92	6.25	2.65	5.31	3.12
private not-for-profit	7.49	2.67	7.07	3.73	7.61	4.89	7.16	6.89
religious not-for profit	7.69	2.44	7.08	2.90	7.50	4.31	6.26	4.43
government not-for-profit	6.81	3.11	6.76	4.84	8.39	8.08	8.73	10.20

*Mean ALOS

registered nurses (RNs) is one method of accounting for a hospital's labor practices. LPNs are nurses who have graduated from an approved school of practical nursing and who work under the supervision of a registered nurse or physician. Generally speaking, a relatively high ratio of LPNs to RNS indicates lower-intensity services than at hospitals with a relatively low ratio of LPNs to RNs.

Researchers have found that teaching hospitals, which generally treat more serious cases, "employ a significantly higher ratio of skilled to licensed practical nurses than do non-teaching facilities."[35] In Table 14, which presents ratios of full-time LPNs to full-time RNs by hospital type, we see that public hospitals have a higher ratio of full-time LPNs to full-time RNs than their counterparts. This finding is consistent with research by Kuhn, Hartz, Gottlieb and Rimm, who found that "public hospitals had a significantly lower proportion of board certified specialists and registered nurses and had higher payroll expenses per bed than private not-for-profit hospitals."[36] The same researchers found that "higher training of medical personnel was very significantly related to lower problem rates and lower adjusted mortality rates."[37]

The Ratio of Technology Services

The ratio of technology services is the final internal variable that is controlled for in the analysis of the relationship between hospital type and hospital efficiency and community service outcomes. Acquisition and utilization of medical technology is costly for hospitals and their communities. In fact, some research indicates that "medical technology may be responsible for as much as 50 percent of the increase in health care spending over the last 20 years."[38] Possessing cutting-edge diagnostics and therapeutic technology, providing innovative practices and participating in research is a definition of excellence that prevails at many hospitals.[39] Among hospitals there is intense competition for patients and physicians - which often entails the use of technology as an inducement for both groups.[40] "Administrators fear that if a certain technology is not available at their facility, physicians would seek affiliations with hospitals where the technology was at their disposal."[41]

In a study analyzing hospitals' acquisitions of magnetic resonance imagers (MRIs), researchers found that the influence of staff physicians is of paramount importance.[42] Hospital CEOs and

Table 14. Ratio of full-time LPNs to full-time RNs by hospital type

Hospital Type	1980		1985		1990		1994	
	*Mean	SD	Mean	SD	Mean	SD	Mean	SD
For-profit	0.34	0.16	0.29	0.15	0.27	0.15	0.23	0.14
Private not-for-profit	0.30	0.15	0.24	0.14	0.21	0.14	0.18	0.13
Religious not-for profit	0.29	0.14	0.22	0.13	0.19	0.13	0.15	0.11
Government not-for-profit	0.40	0.18	0.34	0.17	0.31	0.17	0.28	0.17

*Mean LPN Ratio

boards must depend on physicians' assessment of new technologies because of their access to information about new technologies.[43] Unlike administrators and board members, "physicians enjoy tremendous access to medical information through continuing education, professional journals, and conferences and professional meetings."[44] Hospitals may risk losing physicians and specialists "when they do not provide up to date diagnostic services, are unable to care for certain types of patients or are unable to perform certain surgical and therapeutic procedures. Once a hospital's medical staff starts to send patients to another facility, that hospital suffers a loss of revenue and further deterioration of its ability to maintain 'cutting-edge high technology.'"[45]

The ratio of technology services represents the proportion of the nine surveyed technology services offered by a hospital. Table 15 presents the ratio of technology services by hospital type. As the table shows, private not-for-profit hospitals and religious not-for-profit hospitals have had the highest ratios of technology services over the past fifteen years. By controlling for the availability of technology services at a hospital, the research controls for one aspect of a hospital's modernization. Appendix A provides a detailed explanation of the creation of the technology variable for each year in this study.

Table 16 provides the correlations for the internal hospital-characteristic variables in this analysis.

EXTERNAL FACTORS THAT MAY CONFOUND POSSIBLE EXPLANATIONS OF CONVERGENCE IN THE HOSPITAL INDUSTRY

Previous research has found that environmental factors are significant determinants of hospital strategies. When comparing hospital outcomes, therefore, it is necessary to control for significant environmental factors.[46] That is, the so-called convergence between for-profit and not-for-profit hospitals may actually result from both types of hospitals facing similar environmental factors.

To ensure that the findings are not confounded by external factors, the research controls for hospital environmental factors that previous researchers have found to be significant: hospital location, the hospital market, the ratio of specialists to general practitioners, the proportion of the population who are members of

Table 15. Ratio of technology services according to hospital type

Hospital Type	1980		1985		1990		1994	
	*Mean	SD	Mean	SD	Mean	SD	Mean	SD
for-profit	0.28	0.24	0.30	0.21	0.34	0.24	0.43	0.27
private not-for-profit	0.34	0.30	0.35	0.26	0.38	0.29	0.44	0.30
religious not-for profit	0.48	0.33	0.35	0.26	0.50	0.30	0.56	0.30
government not-for-profit	0.19	0.24	0.23	0.24	0.22	0.26	0.27	0.28

*Mean ratio of technology services

Table 16. Correlations for internal independent variables (2 tailed significant at .01 level **, .05 level *)

1980		1	2	3	4	5	6	7	8	9
1	private not-for-profit hospital	1.000								
2	religious not-for-profit hospital	-0.359 **	1.000							
3	for-profit hospital	-0.323 **	-0.135 **	1.000						
4	government not-for-profit hospital	-0.605 **	-0.254 **	-0.228 **	1.000					
5	hospital has system affiliation	-0.175 **	0.134 **	0.325 **	-0.129 **	1.000				
6	hospital has fewer than 100 beds	-0.142 **	-0.184 **	0.004	0.287 **	0.043 **	1.000			
7	100 to 249 beds	0.071 **	-0.013	0.097	-0.133 **	0.032 *	-0.605 **	1.000		
8	250 to 399 beds	0.068 **	0.142 **	-0.044 **	-0.149 **	-0.058 **	-0.349 **	-0.265 **	1.000	
9	400 or more beds	0.046 **	0.158 **	-0.102 **	-0.097 **	-0.053 **	-0.313 **	-0.238 **	-0.137 **	1.000
10	medical-school affiliation	0.029 *	0.154 **	-0.092 **	-0.083 **	-0.025	-0.254 **	-0.083 **	0.197 **	0.314 **
11	COTH member	0.072 **	0.003	-0.085 **	-0.023	-0.067 **	-0.218 **	-0.145 **	0.027	0.534 **
12	intern or residency program	0.086 **	0.059 **	-0.042 **	-0.109 **	-0.030 *	-0.170 **	0.066 **	0.106 **	0.058 **
13	proportion of operations that are inpatient	-0.085 **	0.019	0.044 **	0.048 **	0.017	-0.026	0.042 **	-0.021	0.002
14	Medicaid ip days as a prop. of adj ip days	-0.020	-0.038 **	-0.009	0.056 **	-0.010	-0.054 **	0.020	-0.010	0.066 **
15	Medicare ip days as a prop. of adj ip days	-0.032 *	-0.006	0.060 **	-0.001	-0.019	0.218 **	-0.106 **	-0.058 **	-0.127 **
16	ratio of full-time LPNs to full time RNs	-0.170 **	-0.088 **	0.019	0.237 **	0.009	0.265 **	-0.021	-0.172 **	-0.204 **
17	average length of stay using inpatient days	0.030 *	0.019	-0.072 **	0.003	-0.026	-0.055 **	0.016	0.015	0.047 **
18	ratio of technology services	0.093 **	0.217 **	-0.033 *	-0.238 **	-0.041 **	-0.630 **	0.000	0.361 **	0.610 **

1985		1	2	3	4	5	6	7	8	9
1	private not-for-profit hospital	1.000								
2	religious not-for-profit hospital	-0.361 **	1.000							
3	for-profit hospital	-0.351 **	-0.142 **	1.000						
4	government not-for-profit hospital	-0.589 **	-0.238 **	-0.232 **	1.000					
5	hospital has system affiliation	-0.148 **	0.224 **	0.258 **	-0.190 **	1.000				
6	hospital has fewer than 100 beds	-0.151 **	-0.175 **	0.011	0.289 **	-0.006	1.000			
7	100 to 249 beds	0.058 **	0.006	0.095 **	-0.138 **	0.025	-0.606 **	1.000		
8	250 to 399 beds	0.083 **	0.117 **	-0.051 **	-0.142 **	-0.024	-0.353 **	-0.277 **	1.000	
9	400 or more beds	0.062 **	0.143 **	-0.106 **	-0.098 **	-0.001	-0.298 **	-0.234 **	-0.136 **	1.000
10	medical-school affiliation	0.058 **	0.160 **	-0.104 **	-0.108 **	0.033 *	-0.264 **	-0.077 **	0.260 **	0.252 **
11	COTH member	0.067 **	0.035 *	-0.090 **	-0.034 *	-0.052 **	-0.231 **	-0.158 **	0.056 **	0.555 **
12	intern or residency program	0.088 **	0.000	-0.024	-0.080 **	0.010	-0.103 **	0.079 **	0.038 **	0.003
13	proportion of operations that are inpatient	-0.133 **	0.005	0.038 **	0.117 **	-0.001	0.005	-0.043 **	-0.021	0.081 **
14	Medicaid ip days as a prop. of adj ip days	-0.023	-0.041 **	-0.096 **	0.126 **	-0.030 *	-0.011	0.068 **	-0.067 **	-0.010
15	Medicare ip days as a prop. of adj ip days	0.027 *	0.039 **	0.035 *	-0.085 **	-0.013	0.048 **	-0.052 **	0.039 **	-0.042 **
16	ratio of full-time LPNs to full time RNs	-0.187 **	-0.121 **	0.046 **	0.264 **	-0.035 *	0.281 **	-0.029 *	-0.177 **	-0.211 **
17	average length of stay using inpatient days	0.007	-0.032 *	-0.080 **	0.074 **	-0.054 **	0.006	0.017	-0.024	-0.008
18	ratio of technology services	0.090 **	0.214 **	-0.026	-0.240 **	0.040 **	-0.634 **	0.042 **	0.370 **	0.547 **

1990		1	2	3	4	5	6	7	8	9
1	private not-for-profit hospital	1.000								
2	religious not-for-profit hospital	-0.360 **	1.000							
3	for-profit hospital	-0.357 **	-0.141 **	1.000						
4	government not-for-profit hospital	-0.590 **	-0.232 **	-0.231 **	1.000					
5	hospital has system affiliation	-0.111 **	0.265 **	0.240 **	-0.247 **	1.000				
6	hospital has fewer than 100 beds	-0.147 **	-0.156 **	-0.039 **	0.308 **	-0.071 **	1.000			
7	100 to 249 beds	0.054 **	0.009	0.129 **	-0.162 **	0.031 *	-0.604 **	1.000		
8	250 to 399 beds	0.081 **	0.116 **	-0.037 *	-0.148 **	0.015	-0.358 **	-0.279 **	1.000	
9	400 or more beds	0.065 **	0.109 **	-0.094 **	-0.084 **	0.052 **	-0.295 **	-0.230 **	-0.136 **	1.000
10	medical-school affiliation	0.065 **	0.163 **	-0.092 **	-0.125 **	0.074 **	-0.296 **	-0.052 **	0.269 **	0.255 **
11	COTH member	0.070 **	0.009	-0.087 **	-0.020	-0.037 *	-0.218 **	-0.147 **	0.044 **	0.537 **
12	intern or residency program	0.062 **	-0.006	0.037 **	-0.092 **	0.029 *	-0.092 **	0.104 **	-0.003	-0.006
13	proportion of operations that are inpatient	-0.021	0.045 **	-0.019	0.004	0.025	-0.211 **	-0.008	0.122 **	0.218 **
14	Medicaid ip days as a prop. of adj ip days	-0.041 **	-0.049 **	-0.096 **	0.152 **	-0.031 *	-0.041 **	0.070 **	-0.069 **	0.039 **
15	Medicare ip days as a prop. of adj ip days	0.035 *	0.069 **	0.109 **	-0.170 **	0.039 **	-0.106 **	0.016	0.120 **	0.011
16	ratio of full-time LPNs to full time RNs	-0.204 **	-0.124 **	0.061 **	0.276 **	-0.089 **	0.339 **	-0.074 **	-0.190 **	-0.222 **
17	average length of stay using inpatient days	-0.009	-0.034 *	-0.083 **	0.096 **	-0.046 **	0.054 **	0.008	-0.065 **	-0.028
18	ratio of technology services	0.119 **	0.200 **	-0.004	-0.277 **	0.113 **	-0.639 **	0.042 **	0.395 **	0.528 **

1994		1	2	3	4	5	6	7	8	9
1	private not-for-profit hospital	1.000								
2	religious not-for-profit hospital	-0.367 **	1.000							
3	for-profit hospital	-0.352 **	-0.131 **	1.000						
4	government not-for-profit hospital	-0.607 **	-0.226 **	-0.217 **	1.000					
5	hospital has system affiliation	-0.062 **	0.236 **	0.216 **	-0.255 **	1.000				
6	hospital has fewer than 100 beds	-0.131 **	-0.146 **	-0.071 **	0.303 **	-0.119 **	1.000			
7	100 to 249 beds	0.042 **	0.017	0.151 **	-0.166 **	0.031 *	-0.606 **	1.000		
8	250 to 399 beds	0.069 **	0.114 **	-0.036 *	-0.135 **	0.063 **	-0.350 **	-0.290 **	1.000	
9	400 or more beds	0.069 **	0.080 **	-0.079 **	-0.080 **	0.073 **	-0.284 **	-0.236 **	-0.136 **	1.000
10	medical-school affiliation	0.101 **	0.129 **	-0.096 **	-0.139 **	0.070 **	-0.285 **	-0.025	0.243 **	0.225 **
11	COTH member	0.068 **	0.002	-0.083 **	-0.019	0.019	-0.215 **	-0.150 **	0.051 **	0.530 **
12	intern or residency program	0.039 *	0.032 *	0.039 *	-0.094 **	0.049 **	-0.129 **	0.094 **	0.057 **	-0.003
13	proportion of operations that are inpatient	0.031 *	0.053 **	0.010	-0.081 **	0.058 **	-0.323 **	0.053 **	0.158 **	0.265 **
14	Medicaid ip days as a prop. of adj ip days	-0.047 **	-0.047 **	-0.039 **	0.115 **	-0.055 **	-0.100 **	0.068 **	-0.017	0.077 **
15	Medicare ip days as a prop. of adj ip days	0.046 **	0.087 **	0.131 **	-0.209 **	0.070 **	-0.172 **	0.052 **	0.139 **	0.040 **
16	ratio of full-time LPNs to full time RNs	-0.204 **	-0.126 **	0.045 **	0.290 **	-0.130 **	0.335 **	-0.081 **	-0.179 **	-0.216 **
17	average length of stay using inpatient days	-0.023	-0.037 *	-0.072 **	0.103 **	-0.068 **	0.061 **	-0.004	-0.051 **	-0.034 *
18	ratio of technology services	0.141 **	0.185 **	0.012	-0.302 **	0.168 **	-0.654 **	0.094 **	0.399 **	0.463 **

Table 16. (Continued)

1980	10	11	12	13	14	15	16	17	18
1 private not-for-profit hospital									
2 religious not-for-profit hospital									
3 for-profit hospital									
4 government not-for-profit hospital									
5 hospital has system affiliation									
6 hospital has fewer than 100 beds									
7 100 to 249 beds									
8 250 to 399 beds									
9 400 or more beds									
10 medical-school affiliation	1.000								
11 COTH member	-0.071 **	1.000							
12 intern or residency program	-0.064 **	-0.054 **	1.000						
13 proportion of operations that are inpatient	-0.029 *	-0.005	0.007	1.000					
14 Medicaid ip days as a prop. of adj ip days	0.031 *	0.139 **	0.036 **	0.015	1.000				
15 Medicare ip days as a prop. of adj ip days	-0.079 **	-0.140 **	-0.032 *	0.023	-0.199 **	1.000			
16 ratio of full-time LPNs to full time RNs	-0.122 **	-0.201 **	-0.052 **	0.111 **	0.056 **	0.124 **	1.000		
17 average length of stay using inpatient days	0.009	0.041 **	-0.001	-0.116 **	0.063 **	-0.347 **	0.011	1.000	
18 ratio of technology services	0.349 **	0.469 **	0.132 **	0.007	0.047 **	-0.155 **	-0.336 **	-0.033 *	1.000
1985									
1 private not-for-profit hospital									
2 religious not-for-profit hospital									
3 for-profit hospital									
4 government not-for-profit hospital									
5 hospital has system affiliation									
6 hospital has fewer than 100 beds									
7 100 to 249 beds									
8 250 to 399 beds									
9 400 or more beds									
10 medical-school affiliation	1.000								
11 COTH member	-0.081 **	1.000							
12 intern or residency program	-0.056 **	-0.048 **	1.000						
13 proportion of operations that are inpatient	0.008	0.062 **	-0.004	1.000					
14 Medicaid ip days as a prop. of adj ip days	-0.054 **	0.042 **	-0.013	0.010	1.000				
15 Medicare ip days as a prop. of adj ip days	0.005	-0.082 **	-0.002	0.087 **	-0.516 **	1.000			
16 ratio of full-time LPNs to full time RNs	-0.122 **	-0.208 **	-0.035 *	0.152 **	0.078 **	0.114 **	1.000		
17 average length of stay using inpatient days	-0.034 *	-0.008	-0.026	-0.132 **	0.459 **	-0.369 **	-0.045 **	1.000	
18 ratio of technology services	0.322 **	0.454 **	0.075 **	0.045 **	-0.145 **	0.054 **	-0.312 **	-0.137 **	1.000
1990									
1 private not-for-profit hospital									
2 religious not-for-profit hospital									
3 for-profit hospital									
4 government not-for-profit hospital									
5 hospital has system affiliation									
6 hospital has fewer than 100 beds									
7 100 to 249 beds									
8 250 to 399 beds									
9 400 or more beds									
10 medical-school affiliation	1.000								
11 COTH member	-0.088 **	1.000							
12 intern or residency program	-0.060 **	-0.042 **	1.000						
13 proportion of operations that are inpatient	0.129 **	0.201 **	-0.008	1.000					
14 Medicaid ip days as a prop. of adj ip days	-0.025	0.088 **	-0.011	0.008	1.000				
15 Medicare ip days as a prop. of adj ip days	0.063 **	-0.059 **	0.025	0.136 **	-0.538 **	1.000			
16 ratio of full-time LPNs to full time RNs	-0.172 **	-0.199 **	-0.023	-0.021	0.125 **	0.025	1.000		
17 average length of stay using inpatient days	-0.054 **	-0.028	-0.027	-0.198 **	0.413 **	-0.365 **	0.006	1.000	
18 ratio of technology services	0.352 **	0.401 **	0.038 **	0.287 **	-0.146 **	0.213 **	-0.388 **	-0.188 **	1.000
1994									
1 private not-for-profit hospital									
2 religious not-for-profit hospital									
3 for-profit hospital									
4 government not-for-profit hospital									
5 hospital has system affiliation									
6 hospital has fewer than 100 beds									
7 100 to 249 beds									
8 250 to 399 beds									
9 400 or more beds									
10 medical-school affiliation	1.000								
11 COTH member	-0.097 **	1.000							
12 intern or residency program	-0.082 **	-0.053 **	1.000						
13 proportion of operations that are inpatient	0.153 **	0.233 **	0.023	1.000					
14 Medicaid ip days as a prop. of adj ip days	-0.009	0.086 **	-0.017	0.053 **	1.000				
15 Medicare ip days as a prop. of adj ip days	0.079 **	-0.017	0.046 **	0.202 **	-0.526 **	1.000			
16 ratio of full-time LPNs to full time RNs	-0.175 **	-0.200 **	-0.084 **	-0.178 **	0.160 **	-0.099 **	1.000		
17 average length of stay using inpatient days	-0.052 **	-0.040 **	-0.039 **	-0.238 **	0.431 **	-0.376 **	0.161 **	1.000	
18 ratio of technology services	0.309 **	0.369 **	0.107 **	0.380 **	-0.143 **	0.294 **	-0.454 **	-0.227 **	1.000

health maintenance organizations, proportion of the population age 65 and over, county per capita income and county unemployment rate. Table 17 presents the means and standard deviations for these environmental variables for each year in the study. Table 18 presents the correlations for each of the environmental variables.

Hospital Location

This analysis controls for two levels of a hospital's location: state location, and whether the hospital is located in an urban or rural area.

State Location

This analysis uses hospitals from every state in the contiguous United States. Using dummy variables to control for state location enables the researcher to control for the variation in the purchasing power of a dollar. Controlling for state location also enables the researcher to control for the absence or presence of certificate-of-need (CON) legislation and state review programs. State CON programs control hospitals' capital expenditures. In states with CON legislation, hospitals are required to have state approval prior to the purchase of specified equipment, construction or expansion.[47] In states with rate-review programs, agencies regulate hospitals' operating revenues.[48] The state dummy variables allowed the researcher to control for the presence or absence of local regulations that may shape operating strategies of specific hospitals. In this research, the state of New York is used as the reference category.

Urban-Rural Location

Other studies discuss the importance of controlling for urban or rural location, because both settings present unique challenges. Hospitals in rural areas generally have trouble attracting and retaining highly skilled staff.[49] Furthermore, rural hospitals generally do not have the capacity to offer the wide array of services available at urban hospitals. Consequently, researchers find that rural hospitals have lower costs than urban hospitals.[50]

By contrast, the situation of urban hospitals apparently leads to relatively high costs. First, urban hospitals face challenges inherent in being located in metropolitan areas with potential patients

Table 17. Means and standard deviations for environmental characteristics

Environmental Variables	1980 (N=4559)		1985 (N=4503)		1990 (N=4315)		1994 (N=3957)	
	Mean	SD	Mean	SD	Mean	SD	Mean	SD
ratio of specialists to generalist MDs	0.169	0.085	0.191	0.087	0.195	0.088	0.207	0.094
5-year change in the MD ratio	0.020	0.049	0.022	0.057	0.003	0.053	0.013	0.056
proportion of population age 65 and over	0.122	0.034	0.128	0.033	0.139	0.037	0.139	0.036
5-year change in the proportion of population age 65+	0.005	0.007	0.007	0.008	0.010	0.009	0.001	0.005
per-capita income (1994 dollars)	15944	3214	17657	3673	19499	4164	19942	4020
5-year change in the per-capita income	0.060	0.078	0.111	0.098	0.105	0.067	0.032	0.059
unemployment rate	7.226	2.573	7.832	2.977	5.765	1.876	6.031	2.053
proportion of population who are HMO members	0.017	0.076	0.046	0.100	0.066	0.119	0.076	0.132
hospital market (Herfindahl Index)	0.414	0.363	0.421	0.366	0.442	0.376	0.466	0.381
urban location	0.510	0.500	0.540	0.500	0.550	0.500	0.560	0.500
rural location	0.490	0.500	0.460	0.500	0.450	0.500	0.440	0.500

Note: The state location of the hospital is controlled for with use of dummy variables.
New York State is used as the reference category.

Table 18. Correlations for environmental variables (Note: 2 tailed significant at .01 level **, .05 level *)

1980	1	2	3	4	5	6	7	8	9	10	11
1 ratio of specialists to generalist MDs	1.000										
2 5 yr chng in MD ratio	0.399 **	1.000									
3 proportion age 65 and over	-0.329 **	-0.009	1.000								
4 5 yr chng in 65+ proportion	-0.002	-0.038 **	0.218 **	1.000							
5 per capita income - 1994 $s	0.377 **	-0.039 **	-0.268 **	0.027	1.000						
6 5 yr chng in income	0.193 **	0.045 **	-0.126 **	-0.103 **	0.216 **	1.000					
7 unemployment rate	0.027	0.066 **	-0.129 **	0.018	-0.285 **	-0.101 **	1.000				
8 proportion HMO members	0.151 **	-0.004	-0.131 **	-0.078 **	0.276 **	0.075 **	-0.040 **	1.000			
9 hosp. mkt./Herfindahl Index	-0.512 **	0.014	0.364 **	-0.017	-0.630 **	-0.185 **	0.060 **	-0.222 **	1.000		
10 urban location	0.467 **	-0.029 *	-0.398 **	0.000	0.588 **	0.159 **	-0.074 **	0.202 **	-0.744 **	1.000	
11 rural location	-0.467 **	0.029 *	0.398 **	0.000	-0.588 **	-0.159 **	0.074 **	-0.202 **	0.744 **	-1.000 **	1.000
1985											
1 ratio of specialists to generalist MDs	1.000										
2 5 yr chng in MD ratio	0.410 **	1.000									
3 proportion age 65 and over	-0.304 **	-0.001	1.000								
4 5 yr chng in 65+ proportion	0.123 **	-0.005	0.016	1.000							
5 per capita income - 1994 $s	0.361 **	-0.045 **	-0.202 **	0.019	1.000						
6 5 yr chng in income	0.061 **	-0.005	0.135 **	-0.068 **	0.296 **	1.000					
7 unemployment rate	-0.125 **	0.021	-0.024	-0.021	-0.528 **	-0.357 **	1.000				
8 proportion HMO members	0.242 **	-0.008	-0.244 **	-0.021	0.438 **	0.050 **	-0.199 **	1.000			
9 hosp. mkt./Herfindahl Index	-0.474 **	0.047 **	0.363 **	-0.079 **	-0.646 **	-0.070 **	0.273 **	-0.420 **	1.000		
10 urban location	0.469 **	-0.040 **	-0.399 **	0.120 **	0.607 **	0.065 **	-0.283 **	0.389 **	-0.786 **	1.000	
11 rural location	-0.469 **	0.040 **	0.399 **	-0.120 **	-0.607 **	-0.065 **	0.283 **	-0.389 **	0.786 **	-1.000 **	1.000
1990											
1 ratio of specialists to generalist MDs	1.000										
2 5 yr chng in MD ratio	0.320 **	1.000									
3 proportion age 65 and over	-0.302 **	0.023	1.000								
4 5 yr chng in 65+ proportion	-0.221 **	0.029 *	0.388 **	1.000							
5 per capita income - 1994 $s	0.328 **	-0.021	-0.186 **	-0.229 **	1.000						
6 5 yr chng in income	-0.048 **	0.033 *	0.147 **	0.245 **	0.134 **	1.000					
7 unemployment rate	-0.020	0.036 *	-0.007	0.012	-0.440 **	-0.100 **	1.000				
8 proportion HMO members	0.256 **	-0.036 *	-0.319 **	-0.258 **	0.471 **	-0.104 **	-0.167 **	1.000			
9 hosp. mkt./Herfindahl Index	-0.457 **	0.017	0.395 **	0.314 **	-0.624 **	0.103 **	0.190 **	-0.495 **	1.000		
10 urban location	0.451 **	-0.018	-0.422 **	-0.293 **	0.570 **	-0.088 **	-0.195 **	0.449 **	-0.800 **	1.000	
11 rural location	-0.451 **	0.018	0.422 **	0.293 **	-0.570 **	0.088 **	0.195 **	-0.449 **	0.800 **	-1.000 **	1.000
1994											
1 ratio of specialists to generalist MDs	1.000										
2 5 yr chng in MD ratio	0.354 **	1.000									
3 proportion age 65 and over	-0.319 **	-0.048 *	1.000								
4 5 yr chng in 65+ proportion	0.080 **	0.000	-0.056 **	1.000							
5 per capita income - 1994 $s	0.316 **	-0.012	-0.166 **	0.251 **	1.000						
6 5 yr chng in income	0.039 **	0.020	-0.038 *	-0.021	-0.007	1.000					
7 unemployment rate	0.114 **	0.070 **	-0.060 **	-0.026	-0.299 **	-0.107 **	1.000				
8 proportion HMO members	0.272 **	0.020	-0.303 **	0.139 **	0.451 **	-0.105 **	-0.064 **	1.000			
9 hosp. mkt./Herfindahl Index	-0.444 **	-0.004	0.392 **	-0.167 **	-0.631 **	0.051 **	0.039 **	-0.533 **	1.000		
10 urban location	0.461 **	0.004	-0.446 **	0.171 **	0.593 **	0.003	-0.077 **	0.490 **	-0.844 **	1.000	
11 rural location	-0.461 **	-0.004	0.446 **	-0.171 **	-0.593 **	-0.003	0.077 **	-0.490 **	0.844 **	-1.000 **	1.000

from varying socioeconomic levels. In recent years, for example, much has been written about overcrowding in inner-city emergency departments.[51] Second, urban hospitals typically offer a wide array of services. They are, for example, more likely to use breast-conserving techniques in preference to mastectomy. Breast conserving techniques require more surgical and radiology facilities than do mastectomies.[52] Research indicates that the presence of these services increases expenses per adjusted admission. In fact, one study estimates that metropolitan hospitals' costs are approximately "eleven percent greater than non-metropolitan hospitals controlling for other factors. These results may reflect geographic differences in unobserved input prices, case mix, or style of care."[53] By using dummy variables to denote state location and urban versus rural location, the research controls for unmeasured differences in practice patterns, quality of care, and case mix.[54]

Hospital Market

Prior studies indicate the importance of controlling for the local hospital market.[55] The Herfindahl Hirschman Index is the most commonly used measure of market concentration - the extent to which a few hospitals dominate local services.[56] Past studies indicate that hospitals that face competition (i.e., low concentration) have higher costs than hospitals in markets with low competition (i.e., high concentration) because competition promotes the provision of more amenities and a higher quality of care.[57]

In the hospital industry, researchers create the Herfindahl Index using either hospital inpatient days or hospital beds; hospital inpatient days were used in the present analysis. Inpatient days are considered a better proxy for hospital utilization than hospital beds. A Herfindahl Index utilizing inpatient days enables one to capture the hospital's actual market share rather than Hospital A's available beds as a share of all beds in Hospital A's market.[58] The Herfindahl Index was created using both measures; there were minimal differences between the two measures. In this analysis the Herfindahl Index ranges from .02 to 1. Hospitals in areas with low market concentration (a large number of hospitals) have a Herfindahl Index approaching .02; those that have no local competitors have a Herfindahl Index of 1. The Herfindahl Index was created for both counties and PMSAs/MSAs. If the hospital is in a PMSA/MSA it was assigned the Herfindahl Index for the PMSA/MSA where it resides rather than the county.

Hospitals with a large number of competitors are more likely to close in response to financial stress. Those with few competitors are more likely to merge or remain in operation despite financial problems. Community officials in areas with low market concentration try to keep financially distressed hospitals in operation. Researchers indicate that "these weakened institutions may not be providing the best services to their communities because their survival may depend on the absence of viable competitors to which patients can turn".[59] *Appendix B*, lists the 25 markets with the lowest concentration index for each year in the study.

Shortell and colleagues found evidence that hospital competition at the local level are significant in determining the types of services hospitals provide.[60] For instance, "both investor-owned and not-for-profit hospitals offer a greater number of alternative services in more highly competitive markets . . . however, when competition is high, investor-owned system hospitals offer less charity care than when competition is low, while the not-for-profit system hospitals show no difference."[61] They also found that "sole community hospitals provide fewer alternative services than hospitals located in multihospital communities provide."[62] Since concentration has implications for hospital expenses and the services hospitals provide, it is important to include it in the analysis; the Herfindahl Index allows the researcher to do so.

Ratio of Specialists to General Practitioners

Researchers have found that the ratio of general practitioners to specialists affects expenses per adjusted hospital admission. Therefore, it is necessary to control for this ratio in the analysis of hospital efficiency and community service outcomes. In general, when physicians of all types are plentiful in a given area, hospitals compete for physicians' patients by increasing amenities for physicians (e.g., acquiring sophisticated equipment).[63] Regarding the ratio of generalists to specialists, studies have shown that "a highly specialized physician population requires the provision of special hospital facilities in order to practice."[64] Hospitals in communities with a high ratio of specialists to general practitioners, then, may duplicate services to attract referrals. A high level of duplication of services in a given area, in turn, may increase hospital expenses per adjusted admission. Moreover, increases in hospital costs may result from an inappropriate utilization of duplicated services.

In addition to controlling for the ratio of specialists to general practitioners, the study also controls for the five-year change in this ratio. This enables the author to analyze hospital efficiency and community service outcomes in conjunction with environmental changes, including changes in the ratio of specialists to general practitioners.

Population Over the Age of 65

In 1965, Title Eighteen, an amendment to the Social Security Act, made all U.S. citizens over 65 eligible for Medicare health insurance regardless of their place of residence, wealth, and health history. Medicare payments have historically provided hospitals with a generous rate of return.[65] In fact, both not-for-profit and for-profit hospitals in Medicare concentrated areas tailor their services to maximize hospital profits. These hospitals are more likely to have post-acute-care (PAC) facilities, which are lucrative for hospitals, because hospitals with PACs discharge patients earlier than hospitals without PACs.[66] However, this practice can lead to a higher rate of infections or complications.

Fennel and Alexander use the size of the over-65 population as an indicator of demand for head cancer and neck cancer treatments. Because this segment of the population is most at risk for contracting these cancers, this indicator functions as an indicator of both demand and supply for cancer-treatment facilities.[67] Hospitals in Medicare-concentrated areas receive similar Medicare payments for hospital services and exhibit similar patient mixes. Therefore, it is important to control for the percentage of the population over 65 in an analyses of hospital affiance and community service outcomes. The study also controls for the five-year percentage change in the population age 65 and over.

County Unemployment Rates and Per Capita Income

Prior studies indicate the importance of controlling for community wealth.[68] Both unemployment rates and per-capita income are indicators of community wealth. Because the majority of the U.S. population pays for medical services with employer-based health insurance, a high unemployment rate may indicate that the local hospital faces high demand for charitable care. Furthermore, "county per capita income accounts for the differences in hospital quality and amenities that reflect the area's level of affluence."[69] Thus, hospitals in areas experiencing substantial decreases in county per-capita income may face increased demands for charitable care. Because hospitals include the costs of treating underinsured and uninsured patients in their expenses per adjusted admission, hospitals that provide substantial charitable care will have higher expenses per adjusted admission than those that do not. Research indicates that for-profit hospitals intentionally locate in affluent areas, which enables them to control their expenses per adjusted admission.[70]

In a study of emergency-department utilization, Tyrance, Himmelstein and Woolhandler found that "the poor and near-poor had higher per capita emergency department expenditures and spent a larger share of their total medical care dollars in emergency departments than did the more affluent."[71] Other research indicates that "many children from low-income families receive much of their primary medical care at hospital emergency-rooms."[72] Therefore, the research controlled for county affluence (as measured by per-capita income) in addition to the unemployment rate. Moreover, the analyses controlled for the five-year change in both per-capita income and the unemployment rate. By doing so, efficiency and community service outcomes can be analyzed in conjunction with changes in community affluence indicators.

Health Maintenance Organizations

Since 1980, the proportion of the population who are members of health maintenance organizations (HMOs), has increased by 400 percent (see Table 17). "HMOs are known to control medical costs by having a lower hospitalization rate than that experienced by the general population."[73] Some evidence indicates that increased price competition resulting from a substantial growth in HMO enrollment has begun to force down hospital prices in many states.[74]

Researchers find that increases in HMO community concentration appear to increase hospital efficiency outcomes. A recent study of 85 of the largest metropolitan areas by the Group Health Association of America found that, in areas where a high proportion of the population belonged to HMOs, the average annual rate of increases in per-admission hospital cost was 8.3 percent.[75] By contrast, hospital costs grew 11.2 percent in areas where 10 percent or less of patients were HMO members. The researchers also report that "during 1993 the average hospital admission cost $1,180 more in areas with less managed care, compared with communities with more managed care."[76] In other words, these slower cost increases were not restricted to HMO patients; they affected the entire community.[77]

A recent *Wall Street Journal* article suggests, however, that cost-saving measures of HMOs are not always in the best interests of the patients. A recent article in *Consumer Reports* explains that "people who join an HMO give up a lot: the ability to choose where and how they are treated; longstanding relationships with their doctors, who may not be part of the HMO; convenient access to care; and sometimes, care that is essential to their health."[28] HMOs constrain the average cost per hospital bed by restricting lengths of hospitalization following surgery; HMOs also control treatment protocols. Two Connecticut HMOs, for instance, recently began to encourage outpatient mastectomies to save on hospital costs.[29] Therefore, hospitals that treat HMO patients must meet HMO demands to ensure future business. Because HMOs continue to influence hospital treatment protocol it is necessary to control for the proportion of the population who are HMO members.

SUMMARY

This chapter discusses the hospital internal characteristics and environmental characteristics controlled for in the analysis of the declining distinction between hospital types. Chapter 5 discusses the methods that were used to perform the analysis.

NOTES

1. See R. E. Herzlinger, and W. S. Krasker, "Who Profits from Nonprofits?" *Harvard Business Review* (1987): 93–105; B. Arrington, and C. C. Haddock, "Who Really Profits from Not-For-Profits?" *Health Services Research* 25 (1990): 291–304.

2. American Hospital Association, *1994 AHA Guide* (Chicago: American Hospital, 1994) Association.

3. C. L. Estes, and J. H. Swan, "Privatization, System Membership and Access to Home Health Care for the Elderly," *Milbank Quarterly* 72 (1994): 277–298.

4. Ibid.

5. Edmund R. Becker, and Frank Sloan, "Hospital Ownership and Performance," *Economic Inquiry* 23 (1985): 23.

6. T. J. Menke, "The Effect of Chain Membership on Hospital Costs," *Health Services Research* 32 (1997): 177–196.

7. See T. Frist, and J. Campbell, "Outlook for Hospitals: Systems are the Solution," *Harvard Business Review* September-October (1981): 132; J. S.

Coyne, "Hospital Performance in Multihospital Systems: A Comparative Study of System and Independent Hospitals," *Health Services Research* 17 (1982): 303–329.

8.   American Hospital Association, *1994 AHA Guide* (Chicago: American Hospital, 1994) Association. "While size is frequently measured by the number of employees, in hospitals size is most typically assessed by the number of beds. . . . Correlations with the size of the staff are not quite as high, as decisions must be made concerning how to categorize volunteer help and doctors affiliated with but not serving in the hospital all the time." See Jeffrey Pfeffer, and Gerald Salanzick, *The External Control of Organizations* (New York: Harper and Row, 1978), 80.

9.   See K.E. Thorpe, "The Use of Regression Analysis to Determine Hospital Payment: The Case of Medicare's Indirect Teaching Adjustment," *Inquiry* 25(1988) : 225;R. Morey, Y. Ozcan, D. Retzlaff-Roberts and D. Fine, "Estimating the Hospital-Wide Cost Differentials Warranted for Teaching Hospitals," *Medical Care* 33)1995):531.

10.   R. M. Kahn, "The Ritziest Hospitals in Town," *Boston Magazine* 88 (1996): 68–73, 115–120.

11.   Frank A. Sloan, Roger D. Feldman, and A. Bruce Steinwald, "Effects of Teaching on Hospital Costs," *Journal of Health Economics* 2 (1983): 1–28; T. W. Grannemann, R. S. Brown, and M. V. Pauly, "Estimating Hospital Costs: A Multiple-Output Analysis," *Journal of Health Economics* 5 (1986): 107–127.

12.   R. Morey, Y. Ozcan, D. Retzlaff-Roberts, and D. Fine, "Estimating the Hospital-Wide Cost Differentials Warranted for Teaching Hospitals," *Medical Care* 33 (1995): 531; General Accounting Office, *Medicare: Indirect Medical Payments are Too High,* Publication GAO/HRD-89-33 (Washington, DC: Government Printing Office, 1989).

13.   Morey et al., "Estimating the Hospital-Wide Cost Differentials," 532.

14.   K. E. Thorpe, "The Use of Regression Analysis to Determine Hospital Payment: The Case of Medicare's Indirect Teaching Adjustment," *Inquiry* 25 (1988): 225).

15.   W. S. Custer, and R. J. Wilke, "Teaching hospital costs: the effect of medical staff characteristics," *Health Services Research* 25 (1991): 831–857; Morey et al., "Estimating the Hospital-Wide Cost Differentials."

16.   L. H. Friedman, and J. Jorgensen, "Physician's Influence on the Decision to Acquire Magnetic Resonance Imagers in Acute Care Hospitals," *International Journal of Technology Assessment in Health Care* 10 (1994): 672.

17.   E. R. Becker and B. Steinwald, "Determinants of Hospital Casemix

Complexity," *Health Services Research* 16 (1981): 453.

18.   The hospital teaching-commitment variables are constructed to represent level of teaching commitment, with COTH membership as the highest level, medical-school affiliation as the second highest level and an internship or residency program as the lowest level of commitment. If a hospital had all three levels of teaching commitment, it was coded '1' for COTH, and '0' for the other two levels of teaching commitment. A hospital without COTH membership but with both a medical-school affiliation and an internship or residency program was coded '1' for the medical school affiliation and '0' for the other two levels. Hospitals without any teaching commitment are the reference category. Other researchers have used the same method of coding. See Frank A. Sloan, and Edmund R. Becker Becker, "Internal Organization of Hospitals and Hospital Costs," *Inquiry* 18 (1981): 224–239.

19.   K. E. Thorpe, "The Use of Regression Analysis to Determine Hospital Payment," 225.

20.   Frank A. Sloan, and Edmund R. Becker, "Internal Organization of Hospitals and Hospital Costs," *Inquiry* 18 1981: 230.

21.   Frank A., Sloan, and Edmund R. Becker, "Cross Subsidies and Payment for Hospital Care," *Journal of Health Politics, Policy and Law* 8 (1984): 660–85.

22.   See E. L. Hannan, A. L. Siu, D. Kumar, H. Kilburn, and M. R. Chassin, "The Decline in Coronary Artery Bypass Graft Surgery Mortality in New York State," *Journal of the American Medical Association* 273 (1995): 209–213.

23.   Rosemary Stevens, In Sickness and In Wealth: American Hospitals in the Twentieth Century (New York: Basic Books, 1989), 328.

24.   J. P. Weiner, B. H. Starfield, N. R. Powe, M. E. Stuart, and D. M. Steinwachs, "Ambulatory Care Practice Variation within a Medicaid Program," *Health Services Research* 30 (1996): 751–770.

25.   P. McNamara, R. Witte, and A. Koning, "Patchwork Access: Primary Care in EDs on the rise," *Hospitals* (1993): 44.

26.   Ibid.

27.   W. O. Cleverly, "Financial and Operating Performance of Systems: Voluntary versus investor-owned," *Topics in Health Care Financing* 18 (1992): 63–73.

28.   In their study of emergency department utilization, Tyrance and colleagues found that "people age 65 and older had the highest absolute emergency department expenditures, . . . but incurred only 1.1 percent of their medical care costs in emergency departments. Conversely, for those younger than age 18, emergency department costs {were lower}

but represented 4.6 percent of their total medical care spending." See P. H. Tyrance, D. U. Himmelstein and S. Woolhandler, "US Emergency Department Costs: No Emergency," *American Journal of Public Health* 86 (1996): 1527–1531.

29.   G. R. Strange, E. H. Chen, and A. B. Sanders, "Use of Emergency Departments by Elderly Patients: Projections From a Multicenter Data Base," *Annals of Emergency Medicine* 21 (1992): 819–824.

30.   Ibid.

31.   B. M. Singal, J. R. Hedges, E. W. Rousseau, A. B. Sanders, E. Berstein, R. M. McNamara, and T. M. Hogan, "Geriatric Patient Emergency Visits Part 1: Comparison of Visits by Geriatric and Younger Patients," *Annals of Emergency Medicine* 21 (1992): 802–807.

32.   American Hospital Association, The AHA Profile of Hospital Statistics (Chicago: American Hospital Association, 1995), Table 4.

33.   The length of stay debate has focused on all aspects of patient care including mothers and their newborns, see P. Braveman, W. Kessel, S. Egerter, and J. Richmond, "Early Discharge and Evidence-based Practice: Good Science and Good Judgement," *Journal of the American Medical Association,* 278 (1997): 334–336; thoracic surgery patients, see R. M. Engelman, "Mechanisms to Reduce Hospital Stays," *Annals of Thoracic Surgery* 61 (1996): S26–S29; and gynecologic surgical patients, see F. M. Abbas, M. B. Sert, N. B. Rosenshein, M. L. Zahyrak, and J. L. Currie, "Prolonged Stays of OB/GYN Patients in the Surgical Intensive Care Unit," *Journal of Reproductive Medicine* 42 (1997): 179–183.

34.   Classen and colleagues indicate that adverse drug events may account for 140,000 deaths per year in the United States. See D. C. Classen, S. L. Pestotnik, E. R. Scott, J. F. Lloyed, and J. P. Burke, "Adverse Drug Events in Hospitalized Patients: Excess Length of Stay, Extra Costs and Attributable Mortality," *Journal of the American Medical Association* 277 (1997): 301–306.

35.   K. E. Thorpe, "The Use of Regression Analysis to Determine Hospital Payment," 225.

36.   E. M. Kuhn, A. J. Hartz, M. S. Gottlieb, and A. A. Rimm, "The Relationship of Hospital Characteristics and the Results of Peer Review in Six Large States," *Medical Care* 29 (1991): 1034.

37.   Ibid., 1036.

38.   C. A. Steiner, N. R. Powe, G. F. Andersen, and A. Das, "Technology Coverage Decisions by Health Care Plans and Considerations by Medical Directors," *Medical Care* 35 (1997): 484; See also J. P. Newhouse, "An Iconoclastic View of Health Cost Containment," *Health Affairs* 12 (1993): 152.

39.   J. Mantil, R. Willett, and W. Sawyer, "Medical High-Technology Assessment and Implementation in A Community Hospital: Nuclear Magnetic Resonance," *Biomedical Instrumentation & Technology* 25 (1991): 289–296.

40.   Ibid.

41.   L. H. Friedman, and J. Jorgensen, "Physician's Influence on the Decision to Acquire Magnetic Resonance Imagers in Acute Care Hospitals," *International Journal of Technology Assessment in Health Care* 10 (1994): 672.

42.   Ibid.

43.   R. Umbdenstock, "The Role of the Board and its Trustees," In *Health Care Administration: Principles and Practices,* ed. L. Wolper and J. Pena Rockville, MD: Aspen Publications, 1987), 51–57.; Friedman, and Jorgensen, "Physician's Influence on the Decision to Acquire Magnetic Resonance Imagers."

44.   Friedman, and Jorgensen, "Physician's Influence on the Decision to Acquire Magnetic Resonance Imagers" 671.

45.   Mantil, Willett, and Sawyer, "Medical High-Technology Assessment and Implementation," 290.

46.   Sloan, and Becker, "Internal Organization of Hospitals and Hospital Costs;" Sloan, and Becker, "Cross Subsidies and Payment for Hospital Care;" Mary L. Fennel, and Jeffrey A. Alexander. "The Effects of Environmental Characteristics on the Structure of Hospital Clusters," *Administrative Science Quarterly* 25 (1987): 485–510.

47.   S. M. Shortell, E. M. Morrison, S. L. Hughes, B. Friedman, J. Coverdill, and L. Berg. "The Effects of Hospital Ownership on Nontraditional Services," *Health Affairs* Winter (1986): 97–111.

48.   Ibid.

49.   K. M. Sandrick, "Inside Track: Rural Medicine-Family Affair," *Hospital & Health Networks* (October 20, 1996): 52.

50.   See S. D. Culler, A. M. Holmes, and B. Gutierrez, "Expected Hospital Costs of Knee Replacement for Rural Residents by Location of Service," *Medical Care* 33 (1995): 1188–209.

51.   D. Andrulis, A. Kellerman, E. Hintz, B. Hackman, and V. Weslowski, "Emergency Departments and Crowding in U.S. Teaching Hospitals," *Annals of Emergency Medicine* 20 (1991): 980–986; K. Grumbach, D. Keane, and A. Bindman, "Primary Care and Public Emergency Department Overcrowding," *American Journal of Public Health* 83 (1993): 372–378.

52.   Mary E. Johantgen, Rosanna M. Coffey, Harris, D. Robert, H. Levy, and J. J. Clinton, "Treating Early-Stage Breast Cancer: Hospital Characteristics Associated with Breast Conserving Surgery," *American Journal of*

Public Health 85 (1995): 1432–34.

53.   T. W. Grannemann, R. S. Brown, and M. V. Pauly, "Estimating Hospital Costs: A Multiple-Output Analysis," *Journal of Health Economics* 5 (1986): 118.

54.   T. J. Menke, "The Effect of Chain Membership on Hospital Costs." *Health Services Research* 32 (1997): 183.

55.   D. F. Vitaliano, "On the Estimation of Hospital Cost Functions." *Journal of Health Economics* 6 (1987): 305–318; K. E. Thorpe, "Why are Urban Hospital Costs So High? The Relative Importance of Patient Source of Admission, Teaching, Competition, and Case Mix," *Health Services Research* 22 (1988): 821–836; Menke, "The Effect of Chain Membership on Hospital Costs."

56.   J. Mann, G. Melnick, A. Bamezai, and J. Zwanziger, "Uncompensated Care: Hospitals' Responses to Fiscal Pressures," *Health Affairs* (1995) 236–270.

57.   Vitaliano, "On the Estimation of Hospital Cost Functions;" K. E. Thorpe, "Why are Urban Hospital Costs So High;" Menke, "The Effect of Chain Membership on Hospital Costs."

58.   J. Zwanziger, G. Melnick, and K. M. Eyre, "Hospitals and Antitrust: Defining Markets, Setting Standards," *Journal of Health Politics, Policy and Law* 19 (1994): 423–447.

59.   G. J. Bazzoli and E. J. Mackenzie, "Trauma Centers in the United States: Identification and Examination of Key Characteristics, " *Journal of Trauma* (1995) : 104.

60.   Shortell and colleagues (1986) define alternative services as including ambulatory care, geriatric care, health promotion and outpatient diagnostic services. See S. M. Shortell, E. M. Morrison, S. L. Hughes, B. Friedman, J. Coverdill, and L. Berg, "The Effects of Hospital Ownership on Nontraditional Services," *Health Affairs* (1986): 97–111.

61.   Ibid., 107.

62.   Ibid., 108.

63.   J. Hadley, and K. Swartz "The Impact of Hospital Costs Between 1980 and 1984 of Hospital Rate Regulation, Competition, and Changes in Health Insurance Coverage," *Inquiry* 26, (1989): 35–47; Menke, "The Effect of Chain Membership on Hospital Costs."

64.   Fennel, and Alexander, "The Effects of Environmental Characteristics," 322.

65.   The Office of the Inspector General at the Department of Health and Human Services surveyed approximately 39 percent of the hospitals in the Medicare system to determine the impact of this legislation. They

found that for-profit hospitals had an average profit margin of 17.9 percent and not-for-profit hospitals had an average profit margin of 14.8 percent. See U.S. Department of Health and Human Services, Office of the Inspector General, *Financial Impact of the Prospective Payment System on Medicare Participating Hospitals* (Washington, DC: U.S. Department of Health and Human Services, 1984). These profit margins would be considered high by most U.S. business firms. See C.Y. Chang and H. P. Tuckman, "The Profits of Not-For-Profit Hospitals," *Journal of Health Politics, Policy and Law* 13 (1988): 547–64.

66.   L. A. Blewett, R. L. Kane, and M. Finch, "Hospital Ownership of Post-Acute Care: Does it increase Access to Post-Acute Care Services" *Inquiry* 32 (1995/1996): 457–67.

67.   Fennel, and Alexander, "The Effects of Environmental Characteristics,"

68.   Becker, and Steinwald, "Determinants of Hospital Casemix Complexity;" Becker, and Sloan, "Hospital Ownership and Performance."

69.   Sloan, and Becker, "Cross Subsidies and Payment for Hospital Care," 669.

70.   E. C. Norton, and D. O. Staiger, "How Hospitals Ownership Affects Access to Care for the Uninsured," *Rand Journal of Economics* 25 (1994): 171–85.

71.   (Tyrance, Himmelstein, and Woolhandler, "US Emergency Department Costs: No Emergency," 1529.

72.   S. T. Orr, E. Charney, J. Strauss, and B. Bloom, "Emergency Room Use by Low Income Children with a Regular Source of Health Care." *Medical Care* 29 (1991): 283.

73.   Hadley, and Swartz "The Impact of Hospital Costs," 38.

74.   Mann, Melnick, Bamezai, and Zwanziger, "Uncompensated Care: Hospitals' Responses to Fiscal Pressures."

75.   These researchers defined areas with high concentrations of HMO patients as those in which HMOs care for 15 percent of all patients or in which the percentage of HMO patients rose more than 10 percent during the decade.

76.   Hospitals & Health Networks, "Human Resources." *Hospitals & Health Networks,* (October 20, 1996): 11.

77.   Ibid.

78.   Consumer Reports Editors, "Can HMOs Help Solve the Health Care Crisis?" *Consumer Reports* October (1996): 28.

79.   Laura Johannes, "More HMOs Order Outpatient Mastectomies," *Wall Street Journal* (November 6, 1996): B1.

CHAPTER 5

Methods

This chapter describes the methods used to analyze claims of a narrowing distinction between hospital types. Specifically, it describes the processes of verifying and merging the American Hospital Association (AHA) data and the Area Resource File (ARF) data. The chapter also describes the methods used to evaluate the hypotheses.

DATA VERIFICATION

The author relied on two national data sets commonly used by researchers. The AHA data are one of the most commonly utilized sources of hospital information; health-services researchers, public-health officials, sociologists and economists use these data on a regular basis and have corroborated the integrity of the annual data. The Area Resource Files, lists environmental and demographic data by the 3248 FIPS (federal information processing standards) county codes.[1] The ARF files are used regularly by health-service researchers, public-health officials, sociologists and economists who have also corroborated the integrity of the data. Before merging the AHA and ARF, various checks to ensure the reliability of both sets of data were performed.

American Hospital Association Data

Three procedures were performed to ensure the validity of the American Association Hospital data. First, data were verified at the aggregate level for each year of the study by comparing the annual numbers from the data set with the *1995 AHA Hospital Statistics.*[2] Second, the data were verified by comparing local hospital characteristics for each of the years in the study with the AHA Guides for 1980, 1985, 1990 and 1994.[3] Finally, over 300 hospitals were telephoned to verify information from the 1994 AHA data set. In each of the study years hospitals that did not perform operations were found. In order to ensure that this was not misinformation, all 289 hospitals listed as performing *zero* surgical operations in the 1994 AHA data set were telephoned. Minimal discrepancies were found between the data in the data set and the conversations with the hospital personnel. The majority of these hospitals were in rural areas and had fewer than 100 beds. The same procedure was performed for the 44 hospitals listed as having *zero* emergency-room visits in 1994. These verification steps did not reveal any discrepancies, thereby, further corroborating the integrity of the AHA data sets.

Area Resource File Data

Before merging the two data sets, checks were also performed on variables in the Area Resource Files file to ensure the integrity of these data. In fact, a number of these variables were verified with secondary data sources. First, the validity of the physician-distribution numbers in the ARF file were checked by comparing the total number of patient care medical doctors (MDs) and general-practice MDs in the ARF with those in the 1995–1996 edition (1994 figures) of *Physician Characteristics and Distribution in the US;* this comparison was performed for all counties in the states of Georgia and New York. No discrepancies were found between the two files. The unemployment figures for each of the years in the study in the ARF file were compared with figures from the *Report on the American Workforce 1997.*[4] Again, there were no discrepancies between the two sources. Finally, the per-capita income figures from the ARF files for each of the study years were compared with the per-capita income figures in the annual statistical abstracts.[5] Once again, no discrepancies between these two files were found. Therefore, with the above verification procedures, the researcher was confident about the integrity of the data.

DATA MERGE

Both the American Hospital Association data and the Area Resource Files utilize FIPS county codes. Therefore, each hospital in the AHA data set was linked with the appropriate environmental and demographic data. The ARF documentation indicates that since implementation of these codes in 1968 there have been changes; therefore, several procedures were performed to identify modifications in the FIPS county codes between 1980 and 1994. No such discrepancies were found.

Once the researcher was satisfied with the validity of the FIPS codes, the county codes that were in primary metropolitan statistical areas (PMSAs) or metropolitan statistical areas (MSAs) were aggregated.[6] PMSAs and MSAs are "comprised of counties with strong social and economic ties to the area's nucleus. The Census Bureaus has identified 267" of these metropolitan areas.[7] Primary metropolitan statistical areas and metropolitan statistical areas often encompass more than one county. For instance, "in 1990 the Pittsburgh PMSA consisted of four counties (Alleghany, Fayette, Washington, and Westmoreland) which together had 2,056,705 residents."[8] Research indicates that, for hospitals located within them, PMSAs and MSAs, provide a more accurate picture of a hospital's environment than does the particular county where the hospital is located. Therefore, the county-level data for counties that are part of a PMSA or MSA were aggregated.

Following the FIPS verification and the PMSA and MSA aggregation, each of the AHA data files were merged with the appropriate ARF information. All hospitals were matched with the appropriate demographic variables by FIPS code. Those hospitals that were in PMSAs or MSAs were matched with PMSA or MSA information; if a hospital was not in a PMSA or MSA, it was matched with FIPS county-level data. Following the merge, the various demographic statistics for many of the PMSAs and MSAs were compared with published statistics. No discrepancies were found.

Following the merge, each of the four years of AHA data were linked with the appropriate demographic data. Therefore, Hospital Y in Minidoka County, Idaho that is not in a PMSA or MSA, was linked with the demographic information (e.g., per-capita income and unemployment rate) for Minidoka County. By contrast, Hospital X in Sedgwick County, Kansas, part of the Wichita,

Kansas MSA in 1980, was linked with the 1980 demographic information for the Wichita MSA rather than the Sedgwick County
demographic information.[9]

HYPOTHESIS TESTING

Following the data merge, there were four separate files of hospital
information and environmental information for every short-term
general hospital at four points in time: 1980, 1985, 1990, 1994.[10] In
other words, there were four panel data sets.[11] For each data set a
standard ordinary least squares (OLS) regression was performed for
each of the four continuous dependent variables (see Chapter 3):
expenses per adjusted admission, FTEs per adjusted census,
emergency-room visits as a proportion of adjusted inpatient days
and outpatient visits as a proportion of adjusted inpatient days.
OLS regression is "a statistical technique for estimating the relationship between a continuous dependent variable and two or
more continuous or discrete independent variables."[12] Using this
statistical technique, the relationship between the efficiency and
community-service outcomes (the dependent variables) and hospital type (the independent variables) could be examined. For each
study year, regressions were run for the four dependent variables
with the hospital type variables while controlling for the internal
and external independent variables specified above.

The variables were identically specified for each year in the
study to ensure that the relationship between the dependent variables and the independent variables could be compared using the
multiple regression coefficients from 1990 to 1994 or from 1980 to
1985. A "multiple regression coefficient measures the amount of
increase or decrease in the dependent variable for a one unit difference in the independent variable, controlling for the other independent variable or variables in the equation."[13] The changing
effects that the independent variables have on the dependent variables were analyzed, by comparing the regression coefficients for
the same independent variables (hospital type) with the same
dependent variables (e.g., expenses per adjusted admission).

To further test the hypotheses, a t-test was used to compare the
relationships between the four categories of ownership. The t-test
enabled the researcher to compare the private not-for-profit, religious not-for-profit and for-profit hospital groups not only with

the government not-for-profit hospitals (the reference category) but also with the other groups (e.g., the for-profit hospital category and the private not-for-profit hospital category).[14] The t-test also enabled the researcher to further analyze the regression results of the effects of hospital ownership on the efficiency and community-service outcomes.

Most research that analyzes the narrowing distinction in the hospital industry focuses on internal factors. Some research uses both internal and environmental factors; however, these researchers frequently neglect the environmental factors affected by policy change. They also use limited time frames or single points in time. Therefore, the study's goal was to push this area of research further by juxtaposing internal and environmental factors, including policy change, to examine claims of a declining distinction between hospital types. Chapter 6 discusses the results of the analyses.

NOTES

1. "The FIPS county codes were established by the National Bureau of Standards, U.S. Department of Commerce, in 1968, and are published in Federal *Information Processing Standards Publication - Counties and County Equivalents of the United States and the District of Columbia.*" See Bureau of Health Professions, *User Documentation for the Area Resource File (ARF)* (Washington D.C.: Office of Research and Planning, Department of Health and Human Services, 1997).

2. The AHA Hospital Statistic Guides, published annually, present annual American Hospital data at the aggregate level.

3. The AHA Guides, also published annually, serve as directories of all U.S. hospitals.

4. The 1997 *Report on the American Workforce* presents annual average unemployment rates for each year in the study. See *Report on the American Workforce* (Washington, D.C.: U.S. Department of Labor, 1997).

5. I converted all dollar figures (i.e., per-capita income, expenses per adjusted admissions) to 1994 dollars using the consumer price index figures from *Report on the American Workforce 1997.* I followed the procedure for standardizing dollar figures in A.B. Binder, *Finding and Using Economic Information: A guide to sources and interpretation* (California: Bristlecone Books, 1993).

6. "An area is defined as an MSA if there is a city with a population of at least 50,000 or if there is an urbanized area of at least 50,000 population

with at total metropolitan population of at least 100,000. In addition to the county containing the central city, an MSA may include additional counties having close economic/social ties to the central county. MSA's comprise entire counties, except for the six New England states, where towns/cities are the units of definition because of the lack of the county governments. Except for this base unit, the same criteria are applied to define MSA's in New England as in the rest of the country. PMSA's generally have a population of one million or more and are composed of one or more counties, except in New England where they are composed of cities and towns." See *User Documentation for the Area Resource File,* 7.

7.   (Hughes 1998).

8.   (Hughes 1998).

9.   The Wichita Kansas MSA includes Sedgwick County, Butler County and Harvey County.

10.   Though the study is quite comprehensive, the data that I used are panel data. In a ideal world, I would have data for every year in the study.

11.   Like all large data sets, "the data set contained some cases that are outlying or extreme. . . When more than two independent variables are included in the regression model, however, the identification of outlying cases by simple graphics means becomes difficult because the single-variable or two-variable examinations do not necessarily help find outliers relative to a multivariable regression model. Some univariate outliers may not be extreme in a multiple regression model, and, conversely, some multivariable outliers may not be detectable in single-variable or two-variable analyses." See John Neter, William Wasserman, and Michael H. Kutner, *Applied Linear Statistical Models* (Homewood, IL: Irwin, 1990), 393. Therefore, those hospitals whose internal characteristic means were higher or lower than the sum of the year of the study, approximately 9% of the population.

12.   D. Knoke, and G. W. Bohrnstedt, *Statistics for Social Data Analysis* (Itasca, Illinois: F. E. Peacock Publishers, Inc., 1994), 263.

13.   Ibid., 271.

14.   J. Cohen, and P. Cohen, *Applied Multiple Regression/Correlation Analysis for the Behavioral Sciences* (London: Lawrence Erlbaum Associates, 1983).

CHAPTER 6
Results and Conclusion

RESULTS

This chapter presents the results of the multiple regression analyses for the four dependent variables. It also discuses the implications of the analyses for the hypotheses regarding the claims of a narrowing distinction in the hospital industry. Tables 19–22 in Appendix C, present the results of the OLS regressions for the four dependent variables: expenses per adjusted admission, FTEs per adjusted census, emergency-room visits as a proportion of adjusted inpatient days and outpatient visits as a proportion of adjusted inpatient days.

This chapter describes these results in detail, specifically the relationship between type of ownership (for-profit, private not-for-profit, religious not-for-profit and government not-for-profit) and each of the efficiency and community-service variables. The significant relationships between the four dependent variables and the internal and external independent variables in the model are also described. Finally, the results of the t-tests used to test the significance of the relationship between the dependent variables and the four ownership categories are discussed.

OLS Regression Results

Expenses Per Adjusted Admission

Figures 1–4 illustrate the results presented in Tables 19–22. Figure 1, graphs the hospital-ownership regression coefficients for the first

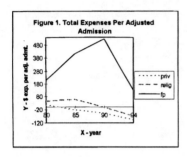

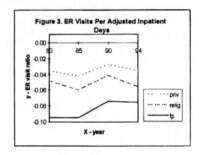

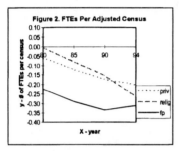

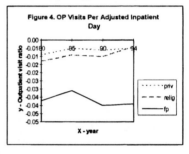

Note: government not-for-profit hospitals comprise the reference category

efficiency dependent variable, total expenses per adjusted admission. Government not-for-profit hospitals were the reference category; therefore, the private not-for-profit, religious not-for-profit and for-profit hospital coefficients are shown in reference to the government category.[1] The X-axis represents years and the Y-axis represents dollars.[2] In 1980, total expenses per admission were approximately $210 (Table 19) higher at for-profit hospitals than at the government not-for-profit hospitals. Figure 1, shows that in 1980 the three hospital types were not in a state of flux. There had been no major federal legislation affecting the hospital industry since the passage of Medicare and Medicaid in 1965.[3] We can also see that in 1980 the for-profit hospitals were playing the reimbursement game better than their not-for-profit counterparts; that is, they were incurring more expenses. Before the passage of the Prospective Payment System, the administrators at for-profit hospitals knew that they would be reimbursed for these expenses. By incurring these extra costs, therefore, they were increasing their bottom line.

We can see that in 1985, following passage of the Prospective Payment System, the legislation that changed the incentive structure in the hospital industry, the various hospital types experimented with different strategies. Chapter 2 summarized neo-institutionalists' description of the uncertainty that organizations face following the implementation of new legislation, and the experimentation that follows in the wake of this new legislation. For instance, in 1985 and, in 1990, the for-profit hospitals were still trying to maximize their bottom lines by incurring higher expenses per adjusted admissions. By contrast, private not-for-profit and religious not-for-profit hospitals were attempting to reduce their expenses in order to work under the newly imposed price controls. By 1994, however, we see that—following the period of experimentation after implementation of the Prospective Payment System—the for-profits and the private and religious not-for-profit hospitals had adopted similar strategies to meet the demands of the cost-containment legislation. This is apparent in the reduction in expenses per adjusted admissions by all three types of hospitals. In fact, "total hospital revenues per case grew by only 5.4 percent in 1993, or 2.4 percent above general inflation—the smallest real increase in more than a decade. Hospitals responded to this pressure by reducing growth in total expenses per case to 5.8 percent."[4]

It is important to reiterate here that Figure 1 is a graph of regression coefficients. These regression coefficients, in turn, are from equations that have controlled for the other explanations, including the local market structure and demographic characteristics of potential patients. Therefore, Figure 1 offers evidence of convergence between not-for-profit and for-profit hospitals. We can see not-for-profit and for-profit hospitals adopting similar strategies that result in similar expenses per adjusted admission. These findings support the first hypothesis that over the past fifteen years, all things being equal, there has been a convergence in the nation's short-term general hospitals as measured by efficiency outcomes.

The regression coefficients for the other internal-characteristic variables and the environmental variables in the model also reveal the expected effects (see Table 19). For instance, compared to the reference category of hospitals with fewer than 100 beds, hospitals with more than 100 beds generally have higher expenses per adjusted admission. There is also a positive relationship between hospitals' teaching commitment and expenses per adjusted admission: consistent with prior research, hospitals that are members of COTH have higher expenses than hospitals with medical-school affiliations and residency and intern programs.[5] The three variables used to control for a hospital's case mix also have a positive effect on hospital expense. The more surgeries a hospital performs, the higher its expenses. And as the literature indicates, those hospitals that treat a higher percentage of Medicaid patients have higher expenses; these patients generally enter the hospital sicker than their counterparts with other types of third-party insurance and are more expensive for hospitals to treat.[6]

The effects of the other internal hospital characteristics were also consistent with prior research. As expected, hospitals with higher ratios of LPNs to RNs had lower expenses per adjusted admission. Substituting lower-paid LPNs for higher-paid RNs enables hospitals to decrease their labor costs.[7] As illustrated by the positive coefficient, hospitals with longer lengths of stay have higher expenses per adjusted admission. Longer lengths of stay are associated with serious complications and illnesses.[8] Finally, the higher the ratio of technology services, the higher the total expenses per adjusted admission. Prior research has shown that it is expensive for hospitals to acquire and maintain the latest technology.[9]

The effects of environmental characteristics on total expenses per adjusted admission were consistent with prior research. For instance, the results indicate that hospitals in urban areas are more expensive than hospitals in rural areas, the reference category. A negative coefficient on the Herfindahl Index indicates that hospitals in areas with lower concentration (generally areas with large numbers of hospitals) have higher expenses than those hospitals in areas with higher hospital concentration (e.g., areas with fewer hospitals). This negative coefficient is consistent with prior research.[10] An increase in the unemployment rate has a positive effect on expenses per adjusted admission. Hospitals in areas with high unemployment are more likely to treat patients without insurance, and therefore to incur higher costs in treating these patients. Ironically, an increase in the per-capita income is also associated with higher expenses per adjusted admission. This finding is consistent with previous findings that for-profit hospitals choose to locate in affluent areas.[11]

Areas with higher proportions of the population age 65 and over have lower expenses per adjusted admission. Hospitals in such areas have fewer patients with other types of insurance coverage on which to shift the expenses of caring for Medicare patients. Some researchers indicate that "rather than controlling costs, hospitals were able to obtain additional revenues to offset Medicare losses. Consequently, the Medicare program is paying less than the costs of furnishing care to its beneficiaries while private payers are paying more."[12] However, hospitals in areas with lower proportions of Medicare patients may not be able to continue their cost-shifting practices. "[P]ayments from private payers as a percentage of patient care costs fell for the first time in 1993, and this trend accelerated in 1994."[13] Therefore, hospitals with relatively few private payers are forced to maintain lower expenses to remain in business in the face of Medicare price controls.

Finally, we see that as the proportion of the population who are HMO members grows (e.g., from 1 percent of the hospital-area population in 1980 to 8 percent in 1994; see Table 17), total expenses per adjusted admission decrease. Many researchers indicate that HMOs constrain hospital utilization for the treatment and care of their patients.[14] Recent findings indicate that average hospital admission costs were lower in areas with high concentrations of HMO patients than in areas with low concentrations.[15]

FTEs per Adjusted Census

Figure 2 graphs the hospital-ownership regression coefficients for the second efficiency dependent variable, full-time-equivalent employees per adjusted census. The year is represented on the X-axis and the number of full-time-equivalent employees per adjusted census on the Y-axis. In 1980 for-profit hospitals had a lower ratio of full-time-equivalent employees per the adjusted census than did government not-for-profit hospitals, the reference category. The trends evident in Figure 2 are similar to those in Figure 1; private not-for-profit, religious not-for-profit and for-profit hospitals have been adopting similar staffing strategies, and they are reducing their medical staffs in an effort to be more efficient. This recent development stands in sharp contrast to the historical pattern, whereby staff reduction strategies were limited to for-profit hospitals.[16] Therefore, graphing the regression coefficients for the second efficiency variable, the number of the full-time-equivalent employees per adjusted census, produces further evidence of convergence between hospital types. In particular, we see that not-for-profits and for-profits are adopting similar strategies in an effort to reduce their labor costs. These findings support the first hypothesis regarding the claims of convergence among short-term general hospitals.

The other internal-characteristic variables in the model for full-time equivalent employees per adjusted census also have the expected effects (see Table 20). The reference category of hospitals with fewer than 100 beds, has fewer FTEs per adjusted census than hospitals with more than 100 beds. Generally speaking, smaller hospitals care for patients with less severe needs than do their larger counterparts.[17] Therefore, these smaller hospitals require smaller medical staffs. Additionally, a teaching commitment has a positive effect on the number of full-time-equivalent employees per adjusted census. As prior research has shown, hospitals with teaching commitments have higher staffing ratios than hospitals that do not have a teaching commitment.[18] In particular, COTH-member hospitals have a significantly higher ratio of FTEs per adjusted census than hospitals with other types of teaching commitments. Case-mix variables have the expected effect on the number of FTEs per adjusted census. The more surgeries a hospital performs, the higher the number of FTEs per adjusted census. As the literature indicates, hospitals that treat a higher percentage of Medicare patients have higher numbers of FTEs per adjusted census. Prior research indicates that Medicare patients utilize more intensive hospital procedures than their younger counterparts.[19] As illustrated by the negative coefficients, hospitals with longer length of stays have lower numbers of FTEs per adjusted census. Government not-for-profit hospitals generally have longer lengths of stay and fewer FTEs per adjusted census. Finally, the higher the ratio of technology services, the higher the number of FTEs per adjusted census. Hospitals that have high ratios of technology services need more personnel to operate and maintain the technology than other hospitals.

The effects of environmental characteristics on the full-time-equivalent employees per adjusted census were also consistent with prior research. For instance, the results indicate that hospitals in urban areas have a higher number of FTEs per adjusted census than hospitals in rural areas, the reference category. Hospitals in urban areas offer a wider array of services, which require more hospital staff, than hospitals in rural areas (Johantgen et al. 1995). The negative coefficient on the Herfindahl Index indicates that hospitals in areas with low concentration (generally urban areas with a large number of hospitals) have higher numbers of FTEs per adjusted census than those hospitals in areas with high hospital concentration (generally areas with few hospitals). This is consistent with the findings for urban hospitals. Finally, we see that as the proportion of the population who are HMO members grows (e.g., from 1 percent in 1980 to 8 percent in 1994; see Table 17), the number of FTEs per adjusted census decreases. Many researchers indicate that HMOs constrain hospital utilization for the treatment and care of their patients.[20] Furthermore, hospitals may be forced to cut their medical staffs as increased price competition from substantial growth in HMOs forces hospital prices down in many states.[21]

Ratio of Emergency-Room Visits per Adjusted Inpatient Day

Figure 3 graphs the hospital-ownership regression coefficients for the first community-service dependent variable, the ratio of emergency-room visits per adjusted inpatient day. The X-axis represents the year, the Y-axis represents the ratio of emergency-room visits per adjusted inpatient day. In 1980, for-profit hospitals had a lower ratio of emergency-room visits per adjusted inpatient day than government not-for-profit hospitals, the reference category.

As we have seen in earlier chapters, many policy analysts and health-services researchers are worried that not-for-profit hospitals are behaving more like their for-profit counterparts and forgoing community service for efficiency. The analysis offers evidence that this is not the case. In 1994, both private not-for-profit and religious not-for-profit hospitals were still providing approximately the same amount of emergency care as they did in 1980. This finding, thus, does not support the notion that private not-for-profit hospitals are becoming more efficient at the cost of community service. Instead we can see that both private not-for-profit and religious not-for-profit hospitals are providing a higher ratio of emergency-room visits than their for-profit counterparts. Furthermore, we can see that private and religious not-for-profit hospitals' provision of charitable care has not been affected by implementation of the Prospective Payment System. In fact, for-profit hospitals were providing slightly more emergency care in 1994 and 1990 than in 1980 and 1985. Some health-service researchers indicate that for-profit hospital administrators have begun to view emergency departments as a loss leader, producing inpatient admissions that will enable hospitals to increase their occupancy rates.[22] However, one could conclude that the emergency departments of for-profit hospitals have limited offerings to those of private and religious not-for-profit hospitals. From graphing the regression coefficients of the ratio of emergency-room visits per adjusted inpatient day (Figure 3), we see that there is no evidence that not-for-profits are reducing their provision of emergency care in an effort to be more profitable. Instead we find that their ratios of emergency-room visits have been relatively stable. These findings do not support the first hypothesis: the evidence does not show a convergence in the nation's short-term general hospitals as measured by the ratio of emergency-room visits per adjusted inpatient day.

The other internal-characteristic and environmental variables in the model for the ratio of emergency-room visits per adjusted inpatient day have the expected effects (see Table 21). Hospitals with fewer than 100 beds, the reference category, have a higher ratio of emergency-room visits per adjusted inpatient day than do the three categories of hospitals with more than 100 beds. In general, there was not a significant relationship between the three case-mix indicators and the ratio of emergency-room visits per adjusted inpatient day. On the other hand, both the average length of stay and the ratio of technical services exhibited a significant relationship with emergency-room visits per adjusted inpatient day. An increase in the average length of stay had a negative effect on the ratio of emergency-room visits. Hospitals with longer lengths of stay treat more serious patients; this relationship indicates that hospitals treating more serious cases are not providing a significant amount of emergency-room care. This finding also explains the lack of a significant relationship between teaching commitment and the ratio of emergency-room visits. For the most part, hospitals with teaching commitments treat more serious cases than hospitals without teaching commitments.[23] A significant relationship was also found between a hospital's ratio of technology services and its ratio of emergency-room visits per adjusted inpatient day; hospitals that have a higher proportion of technology services and facilities provide less emergency care. Once again, we see that hospitals that care for more serious patients are providing less emergency care, indicating that the ratio of technology services and community service are inversely related.

The effects of the environmental variables on the ratio of emergency-room visits per adjusted inpatient day were as expected.

A high proportion of the population aged 65 and over has a negative effect on emergency-room utilization. This finding is consistent with previous studies indicating that people aged 65 and over seek emergency-room care at a lower rate than other sectors of the population.[24] A positive relationship was also found between the unemployment rate and the ratio of emergency-room visits per adjusted inpatient day. This finding is intuitive: people will make more demands on the emergency department as the unemployment rate in a hospital market increases and people lose their insurance coverage. Research has established that emergency rooms are frequent sources of care for those without access to regular health care.[25]

Ratio of Outpatient Visits per Adjusted Inpatient Day

Figure 4 graphs the hospital ownership regression coefficients for the second community-service dependent variable, the ratio of outpatient visits per adjusted inpatient day. The X-axis represents the year and the Y-axis represents the ratio of outpatient visits per adjusted inpatient day. In 1980, for-profit hospitals had a lower ratio of outpatient visits per adjusted inpatient day than government not-for-profit hospitals, the reference category. Outpatient visits are a proxy for the hospital's accessibility to the public. A disproportionate number of a hospital's outpatient services, including screenings and crisis counseling, are used by a disproportionate number of the under- or uninsured.

In 1994 private and religious not-for-profit hospitals were providing substantially more outpatient care than their for-profit counterparts. Figure 4 reveals trends similar to those in Figure 3, which illustrates the ratio of emergency-room visits. It is evident that not-for-profit hospitals are not abandoning their community-service mission as they pursue efficiency strategies. Therefore, these findings do not support the first hypothesis: there is no evidence that the nation's short-term general hospitals are converging as measured by the ratio of outpatient visits per adjusted inpatient day.

Once again, the internal variables had the expected effects. Hospital size has a significant negative relationship with the ratio of outpatient visits; in other words, hospitals with fewer than 100 beds provide a larger ratio of outpatient care than hospitals with more than 100 beds. As we saw in Chapter 3, outpatient care is typically less intensive than other types of hospital services; outpatient services are generally time-consuming and have low profit margins.[26] The negative relationship between hospital size and the ratio of outpatient visits per adjusted inpatient day is consistent with the negative relationship between a hospital's teaching commitment and the ratio of outpatient visits per adjusted inpatient day in the later years of the study (1990 and 1994). Prior to passage of the Prospective Payment System legislation in 1980, there was a positive relationship between a hospital's teaching status and the ratio of outpatient visits. It was not uncommon for teaching hospitals to provide outpatient clinics. By 1990 and 1994, however, there was a negative relationship between a hospital's teaching status and the ratio of outpatient visits.

Furthermore, we can see a negative relationship between the case-mix indicators and the ratio of outpatient visits. Once again, hospitals that treat patients with more serious conditions provide a lower amount of outpatient care. This finding is supported by the negative relationship between the proportion of inpatient operations and the ratio of outpatient visits. Typically, in short-term general hospitals, the most lucrative services are admissions for surgical procedures. While this has been changing in recent years as outpatient ambulatory surgical centers proliferate, surgical inpatients are still more desirable from an organizational and revenue standpoint than outpatient visits. Thus, a hospital with a high ratio of outpatient days to total adjusted days is probably not optimizing its inpatient facilities fully, but is serving a wide range of patient concerns; it is willingly tolerating the inconvenience and difficulties that arise in daily scheduling and allocating resources to less intensive and profitable services. This finding provides support for the negative relationship between outpatient visits per adjusted inpatient day and the average length of stay. In other words, hospitals that have a higher ratio of outpatient visits per adjusted inpatient day have shorter average lengths of stay, indicating a less serious case mix. This relationship is further supported by the negative relationship between the ratio of technology services and the ratio of outpatient visits per adjusted inpatient day. Hospitals with higher ratios of technology services provide less outpatient care than hospitals that have lower ratios of technology services.

Once again, the effects of environmental factors on the ratio of outpatient visits per adjusted inpatient days were consistent with prior findings. In 1980 and 1985, we can see, an increase in the local unemployment rate increases demand for outpatient care. This relationship is consistent with findings from other research indicating that outpatient care is used by those with Medicaid insurance and those without other third-party insurance-an outcome of being unemployed.[27] Interestingly, a negative relationship is apparent between the proportion of the population who are HMO members and the ratio of outpatient visits per adjusted inpatient day. This relationship supports findings from other research indicating that HMOs are attempting to minimize hospital utilization.[28]

T-Test Results

Using the t-test, the second hypothesis can be tested: As financial risk in the health-care industry has increased, hospital type (private not-for-profit, religious not-for-profit, government not-for-profit and for-profit) will be less significant in explaining variation in both efficiency and community-service outcomes in recent years than in previous years.

The results of the four OLS regressions for each year in the study reveal a convergence among short-term general hospitals as measured by efficiency outcomes. By contrast, there has not been a convergence among short-term general hospitals as measured by community-service outcomes. However, OLS regression only enables one to compare categorical differences, in this case ownership type against the reference category, government not-for-profit hospitals. By using the t-test, private not-for-profit, religious not-for-profit and for-profit hospitals can be compared not only with government not-for-profit hospitals (the reference category) but also with each of the other groups.[29]

By analyzing the results of the t-tests (see Table 23) for the hospital-ownership regression coefficients of the efficiency outcomes (expenses per adjusted admission and FTEs per adjusted census), we see that the relationships between the for-profit and religious not-for-profit hospitals are significant. Additionally, we see that the relationship between the private not-for-profit hospitals and the for-profit hospitals is also significant. These significant findings support the graphs of the regression coefficients (Figures 1 and 2) that indicate a convergence between the three hospital types using efficiency outcomes.

Furthermore, we also find support for hypothesis 1a when we look at the changes in the magnitude of the effect of the t. For instance when we compare the magnitude of the effect of the t's from 1980 to 1985 for the expenses per adjusted admission we see that the magnitude of the effect of the t increases and continues to increase from 1985 to 1990. We see that the magnitude of the effect of the t decreases from 1990 to 1994 as the hospital regulatory environment becomes more stable.

Therefore, we find support for the second hypothesis, that as financial risk in the hospital industry increases, ownership type will explain less of the variance in the efficiency outcomes. However, using t-tests, we see that there are significant relationships among the three hospital types for each of the years in the study for the community service variables. The significant relationships among these ownership categories support the graphs of the regression coefficients for the community-service outcomes. Once again, we do not find evidence to support hypothesis 1a with regard to the community-service outcomes. In fact, we find that as financial risk in the hospital industry has increased, (i.e., after the implementation of PPS) hospital ownership type is still significant in explaining the variation in community-service outcomes. With respect to the magnitude of the effect of the t's, we see a slight decrease when we compare the magnitude of the effect of the t's from 1980 to 1985 for both indicators of community service. This decrease in the magnitude of the effect of the t continues when we compare 1985 and 1990 and when we compare 1990 to 1994 for each of the ownership groups. This slight decrease in the magnitude of the regression coefficients further supports the findings that ownership is still significant in explaining the variation in community service outcomes. Table 23, in Appendix C presents the findings for the t-tests.

CONCLUSION AND POLICY IMPLICATIONS

Chapter 1 described the warnings of Paul Starr and other researchers: that, as not-for-profit hospitals have begun to behave like their for-profit counterparts, and as a result, they will abandon their missions of community service in exchange for efficiency. This analysis empirically tested these claims using data for every short-term general hospital in the contiguous states from 1980 to

1994. Additionally, neo-institutional theory is used as a framework for analyzing this question. In this section of Chapter 6, the implications of the findings of the research for neo-institutional theory and United States health care policy are discussed. This section concludes with a brief discussion of future research questions.

Implications For Neo-Institutional Theory

The present findings are consistent with neo-institutional theory. In particular, evidence is found to support the three mechanisms of neo-institutional theory; coercive isomorphism, mimetic isomorphism and normative isomorphism.

In chapter two, the author explained that neo-institutionalists indicate that coercive isomorphism occurs when regulatory changes often force different types of organizations to pursue similar strategies, that, result in similar organizational outcomes.[30] The 1983 Prospective Payment System legislation marked the first time in the history of the hospital industry that hospitals were faced with proscriptive rather than prescriptive legislation. Following the passage of PPS, hospitals were forced to accept price controls, but given little instruction about how to work under these price controls.

Neo-institutionalists explain that organizations experiment with various strategies as they attempt to meet the demands of new legislation: "One possibly desirable effect of the policy change has been to give stronger incentives for hospitals to eliminate unnecessary expense and unnecessary days in the hospital. However, other responses aimed at reducing financial risk might result in reduced patient access to appropriate care."[31] Figures 1 and 2, the graphs of the efficiency coefficients, offer evidence that not-for-profit hospitals have imitated their for-profit counterparts in the pursuit of strategies that result in similar efficiency outcomes. Therefore, one could conclude that passage of the Prospective Payment System legislation prompted the private and religious not-for-profit hospitals to pursue efficiency strategies. Prior to the passage of this legislation not-for-profit hospitals had little incentive to reevaluate their current strategies and look for more efficient ways to provide patient care, because Medicare and other third party insurance payors were reimbursing hospitals for virtually all the costs incurred for an episode of patient care. This finding is consistent with recent work by neo-institutionalists who suggest that efficiency is shaped by the regulatory environment. That is firms do not entertain certain efficiency solutions until policy change occurs.[32]

Neo-institutionalists refer to imitative responses to uncertainty as mimetic isomorphism.[33] In the five years prior to the passage of the Prospective Payment System legislation, policy makers had become alarmed at rising health care costs. Therefore, the hospitals perceived as successful were those with low operating costs. In this analysis there is evidence that mimetic isomorphism occurred following the passage of the Prospective Payment System. In fact, for the first time we see private and religious not-for-profit hospitals adopting efficiency strategies that were once limited to for-profit hospitals. For example, we find many private and religious not-for-profit hospitals reducing their medical staff in an effort to be more efficient. These staff reduction strategies were historically limited to for-profit hospitals.[34]

Finally, neo-institutionalists explain that normative isomorphism is organizational convergence generated by professionals and professional associations. In other research analyzing the hospital industry, evidence is found for normative isomorphism. In fact, using a representative sample of California hospital administrators from 1960 to 1995, the author and a colleague examine whether not-for-profit and for-profit hospitals have converged in the types of administrators that they respectively hire. The research indicates that, in the mid- to late-1960s, not-for-profit hospitals were more likely than for-profit hospitals to hire administrators with medical backgrounds. This difference, however, faded in the 1970s and 1980s—as subsequent federal rulings redefined the charity obligations of not-for-profit hospitals and the pricing procedures of all hospitals.[35] The evidence that the author finds for coercive and mimetic isomorphism in this research and for normative isomorphism in other research supports the hypotheses regarding the convergence among not-for-profit and for-profit hospitals in terms of efficiency outcomes.

Alternately, when the researcher assessed the convergence in hospital types using the graphs of the ownership coefficients for community-service (figures 3 and 4), there is little evidence to support the claims that hospitals are reducing community care in an effort to reduce their expenses. In fact, over the fifteen-year period in this analysis, the not-for-profits and the for-profits have not converged in their provision of community service. This finding is not consistent with neo-institutional theory and leaves many questions unanswered? Why would convergence between these two hospital types occur in terms of efficiency but not in terms of community service? Some may hypothesize that community service is tightly coupled with a hospital's mission. In fact, the mission statement of many private not-for-profit hospital's specifically mentions a hospital's responsibility to their community. These private not-for-profit and religious not-for-profit hospitals have boards that are composed of prominent community members. For-profit hospital boards, on the other hand, are smaller than not-for-profit boards and are often composed of fewer leaders from the hospital community than their not-for-profit counterparts. In subsequent research the author plans to analyze the role of organization missions and hospital boards and the hospital's provision of community service.

From this analysis we can see that there is little evidence that hospitals must choose between efficiency and community service. In fact, the findings from this study indicate that private not-for-profits can simultaneously pursue both efficiency and community service strategies.

U.S. Health Policy Implications

Why should we examine claims of convergence in the hospital industry? Why do we care if for-profit and not-for-profit hospitals have similar expenses per adjusted admission? Prior research indicates that a possible convergence in the hospital industry has many policy implications. As we saw in Chapter 2, all not-for-profit hospitals receive the same property and revenue tax exemptions, regardless of their location, since the passage of the 1969 revenue ruling. Not-for-profit hospitals in rich urban areas, for example, receive the same exemptions as not-for-profit hospitals in poor urban areas. Recent research estimates the resulting tax benefits in billions of dollars.[36] Critics question whether it is cost effective for communities and all levels of government (i.e., local, state and federal) to continue to support hospitals through tax exemptions. Many critics insist that not-for-profit hospitals should not be eligible for tax exemptions if indeed a convergence is occurring in the hospital industry. Others argue that we should not discontinue the exemption; instead hold hospitals accountable for their actions. They suggest penalizing hospitals that are not responsible.

In recent months, the community responsibilities of not-for-profit hospitals have received national media attention. For the first time, "cornerstone" not-for-profit hospitals are merging with for-profit hospitals and other types of for-profit health care organizations. Not-for-profit hospitals—including teaching and church-affiliated—also are being sold to for-profit hospital companies.[37] A recent *Wall Street Journal* article reports that proceeds from the sale of a not-for-profit hospital to a for-profit hospital company were channeled into a newly founded community foundation. Furthermore, money from this foundation has made pilot training a free elective at the local high school. In other communities, sales from not-for-profit hospitals support symphonies and French lessons.[38] One may ask: should this money instead be reinvested in medical services for the community? At present, little legislation regulates the use of proceeds from the sale of these community assets.

In recent years, not-for-profit hospitals have come under fire. Policy analysts question what communities receive for their investments in the form of property and revenue exemptions. Unfortunately, policy makers have few longitudinal studies and nationally comprehensive studies with which to answer these questions.[39] Furthermore, most of the studies that do exist have limited geographic scopes. Therefore, it is difficult for policy makers to use this research to help shape national policy.

Research indicates that the environments in which organizations operate are more definitive than what the institutions call themselves on their legal charters.[40] Yet most researchers do not consider hospitals' environments in their analyses of perceived convergence. Ironically, the hospital environment has become increasingly complex. An increase in the number of hospital mergers and the growth of managed-care organizations and hospital networks are among the factors that contribute to this complexity.

The research analyzes the hypotheses of convergence between not-for-profit and for-profit hospitals in the context of both internal and environmental factors, including the effects of one significant piece of federal legislation, the Prospective Payment System. The research also covers a fifteen-year period. Its scope thus enables me to begin to assess the presence or absence of convergence in the hospital industry.

There is little evidence that not-for-profit hospitals are abandoning their community-service missions as they become more efficient. However, that legislation is necessary to keep private and religious not-for-profit hospitals on the so-called "community service path" as they face increasing cost-containment pressures from their internal and external environments. This is consistent with the researchers who argue that the private and religious not-for-profit sector traditionally has provided and continues to provide community service defined as charity care, losses from public programs, and the costs of teaching and research.[41]

Altman and Shactman explain that without the private and religious not-for-profit sector, "we would become far more dependent on government-run institutions to maintain the health care safety net. As the market-place becomes more competitive, private not-for-profit hospitals preclude the development of a two tiered system—private hospitals for the rich and government hospitals for everyone else."[42] Therefore, legislation holding the private not-for-profit sector accountable to communities would mean wiser use of taxpayer dollars in the health-care arena. Perhaps the days of poorly spent community dollars and federal tax breaks will come to an end: for instance, perhaps there will be no more unnecessary duplication of hospital services and extravagant hospital architecture.

NOTES

1. Hardy specifies that the "reference group should be well defined" and "should contain a sufficient number of cases to allow a reasonably precise estimate of the subgroup mean." See M. Hardy, *Regression with Dummy Variables*, Sage University Paper series on Quantitative Applications in the Social Sciences, 07-093, (Newbury Park, CA: Sage, 1993), 10. In each year of the study, government not-for-profit hospitals represent the second-largest group, following the private not-for-profit hospitals.

2. All dollar figures have been standardized to 1994 dollars.

3. In 1972, the HMO Act marked the beginning of managed care and managed competition in the health-care industry. The National Health Planning Act was passed in 1974. The objective of this legislation was to implement cost containment at the regional level. Finally, in 1978, President Carter "proposed hospital cost containment legislation with prospective limits on each hospital's total revenue increase. The legislative proposal was defeated, with the hospital industry committing to a 'voluntary effort' to control costs. The industry victory was in name only, and the inflation resumed its heated pace." See S. H. Altman, and D. A. Young, "A Decade

of Medicare's Prospective Payment System—Success or Failure?" *Journal of American Health Policy* March/April (1993): 11.

4. S. Guterman, J. Ashby, and T. Greene, "Hospital Cost Growth Down: Unprecedented Cost Constraint by Hospitals has Maintained their Bottom Line. But Can it Continue?" *Health Affairs* 15 (1996): 136.

5. K. E. Thorpe, "The Use of Regression Analysis to Determine Hospital Payment: The Case of Medicare's Indirect Teaching Adjustment," *Inquiry* 25 (1988): 219–231.

6. P. McNamara, R. Witte, and A. Koning, "Patchwork Access: Primary Care in EDs on the rise," *Hospitals* (1993): 44–46.

7. S. Woolhandler and D. U. Himmelstein, "Costs of care and administration at for-profit and other hospitals in the United States," *The New England Journal of Medicine* 336 (1997): 769–74.

8. See R. M. Engelman, "Mechanisms to Reduce Hospital Stays," *Annals of Thoracic Surgery* 61 (1996): S26—S29; F.M.Abbas, M. B. Sert, N. B. Rosenshein, M. L. Zahyrak, and J. L. Currie, "Prolonged Stays of OB/GYN Patients in the Surgical Intensive Care Unit," *Journal of Reproductive Medicine* 42 (1997): 179–183.

9. C. A. Steiner, N. R. Powe, G. F. Andersen, and A. Das, "Technology Coverage Decisions by Health Care Plans and Considerations by Medical Directors," *Medical Care* 35 (1997): 472–489; J. P. Newhouse, "An Iconoclastic View of Health Cost Containment," *Health Affairs* 12 (1993): 152.

10. See T. J. Menke, "The Effect of Chain Membership on Hospital Costs," *Health Services Research* 32 (1997): 177–196.

11. E. C. Norton, and D. O. Staiger, "How Hospitals Ownership Affects Access to Care for the Uninsured," *Rand Journal of Economics* 25 (1994): 171–85.

12. Altman, and Young, "A Decade of Medicare's Prospective Payment System," 18.

13. S. Guterman, J. Ashby, and T. Greene, "Hospital Cost Growth Down," 138.

14. J. Hadley, and K. Swartz, "The Impact of Hospital Costs Between 1980 and 1984 of Hospital Rate Regulation, Competition, and Changes in Health Insurance Coverage," *Inquiry* 26 (1989): 35–47.

15. Hospitals & Health Networks, "Human Resources." *Hospitals & Health Networks,* October 20 (1996): 11.

16. E. A. Sorrentino, "Hospital Mission and Cost Differences," *Hospital Topics* 67 (1989): 22–25; S. Woolhandler and D. U. Himmelstein, "Costs of care and administration."

17.   Rosemary Stevens, In Sickness and In Wealth: American Hospitals in the Twentieth Century (New York: Basic Books, 1989).

18.   R. Morey, Y. Ozcan, D. Retzlaff-Roberts, and D. Fine, "Estimating the Hospital-Wide Cost Differentials Warranted for Teaching Hospitals," *Medical Care* 33 (1995): 531–532.

19.   G. R. Strange, E. H. Chen, and A. B. Sanders, "Use of Emergency Departments by Elderly Patients: Projections from a Multicenter Data Base," *Annals of Emergency Medicine* 21 (1992): 819–824.

20.   J. Hadley, and K. Swartz, "The Impact of Hospital Costs."

21.   J. Mann, G. Melnick, A. Bamezai, and J. Zwanziger. "Uncompensated Care: Hospitals' Responses to Fiscal Pressures," *Health Affairs* (1995): 236–270.

22.   C. G. Homer, D. D. Bradham, and M. Rushefsky, "To the Editor, Investor-Owned and Not-For-Profit Hospitals: Beyond the Cost and Revenue Debate," *Health Affairs* (1984): 133–136.

23.   K. E. Thorpe, "The Use of Regression Analysis to Determine Hospital Payment: The Case of Medicare's Indirect Teaching Adjustment," *Inquiry* 25 (1988): 219–231.

24.   P. H. Tyrance, D. U. Himmelstein, and S. Woolhandler, "US Emergency Department Costs: No Emergency," *American Journal of Public Health* 86 (1996): 1527–1531.

25.   G. L. Albrecht, D. Slobodkin, and R. J. Rydman, "The Role of Emergency Departments in American Health Care," *In Research in the Sociology of Health Care,* ed. J. J. Kronenfeld, (Greenwich, CT: JAI Press, 1996), 289–318.

26.   S. M. Shortell, "The Evolution of Hospital Systems: Unfulfilled Promises and Self-Fulfilling Prophesies," *Medical Care Review* 45 (1988): 177–213.

27.   E. J. Goodwin, et al. "Access to Health Care: Medicare and the Poor Elderly," In *Poverty and Health in the United States,* ed. M. I. Krasner, (New York: United Hospital Fund, 1989); L. K. Abraham, *Mama Might Be Better Off Dead: The Failure of Health Care in America* (Chicago: The University of Chicago Press, 1993).

28.   Hadley, and Swartz, "The Impact of Hospital Costs."

29.   J. Cohen, and P. Cohen, Applied Multiple Regression/Correlation Analysis for the Behavioral Sciences (London: Lawrence Erlbaum Associates, 1983).

30.   N. Fligstein, "The Spread of the Multidivsional Firm, 1919–79." *American Sociological Review* 50 (1985): 377–391; N. Fligstein, "The Structural

Transformation of American Industry: An Institutional Account of the Causes of Diversification in the Largest Firms, 1919–1979." In *The New Institutionalism in Organizational Analysis*, ed. W. W. Powell and P. J. DiMaggio, (Chicago: The University of Chicago Press, 1991), 311–336.

31.   B. Friedman, and D. Farley, "Strategic Responses by Hospitals to Increased Financial Risk in the 1980s." *Health Services Research* 30 (1995): 468.

32.   (see Scott 1995; Scott and Christensen 1995)

33.   P. J. DiMaggio, and W. W. Powell. "The Iron Cage Revisited: Institutional Isomorphism and Collective Rationality in Organizational Fields," *American Sociological Review* 48 (1983): 147–60.

34.   E. A. Sorrentino, "Hospital Mission and Cost Differences," *Hospital Topics* 67 (1989): 22–25; S. Woolhandler, and D. U. Himmelstein, "Costs of care and administration at for-profit and other hospitals in the United States," *The New England Journal of Medicine* 336 (1997): 769–74.

35.   Sharyn J. Potter and Timothy J. Dowd. "Executive Turnover and Strategic Reorientation: the Impact of Ownership Conversion among California Hospitals, 1960-1995." Under Review.

36.   Fox, D. M. and D. C. Schaffer, "Tax Administration as Health Policy: Hospitals, the Internal Revenue Service and the Courts." *Journal of Health Politics, Policy and Law* 16 (1991): 251–279; Nancy Kane, "Report on the Financial Resources of Major Hospitals in Boston." (Department of Health and Hospitals: Boston, 1993).

37.   Sandy Lutz, "Not-For-Profits up for Grabs by the Giants: Teaching, Church-Affiliated Hospitals Ponder Deals with Investor-Owned Firms," *Modern Healthcare* (1994): 24–30.

38.   Greg Jaffe, and Monica Langley, "Generous to a Fault? Fledgling Charities Get Billions from the Sales of Nonprofit Hospitals," *Wall Street Journal* (November 6, 1996.): A1.

39.   Chang and Tuckman, "The Profits of Not-For-Profit Hospitals," *Journal of Health Politics, Policy and Law* 13 (1988): 547–64. Nancy Kane, "Report on the Financial Resources of Major Hospitals in Boston."

40.   Theodore R. Marmor, Mark Schlesinger, and Richard W. Smithey, "Nonprofit Organizations and Health Care," In *The Nonprofit Sector: A Research Handbook*, ed. W. W. Powell, (New Haven, CT: Yale University Press, (1987), 221–240.

41.   Altman, and Young, "A Decade of Medicare's Prospective Payment System."

42.   Altman, and Young, "A Decade of Medicare's Prospective Payment System," 979.

Creation of Hospital Technology Variable

The ratio of technology services, one of the internal hospital characteristics that is used in the research, was calculated using the frequency of technology services and facilities available for each year in the study. The ratios are made up of different facilities and services as new technologies are acquired by hospitals. Therefore, the ratio of technology services is comprised of slightly different technologies in 1980 than in 1994. Table A1 shows the number and percentage of hospitals offering each service for each of the years in the study.

Table A1. Ratio of technology services, 1980–1994

Facility or Service	1980 N	1980 %	1985 N	1985 %	1990 N	1990 %	1994 N	1994 %
Radiation therapy*[1]	1425	31	1315	29	1333	31	1097	28
Computerized tomography scanners	1067	23	2679	59	3254	75	3371	85
Diagnostic radioisotope facility	3150	69	3300	73	2909	67	2490	63
Electromyography	1658	36						
Cardiac catheterizations	741	16	871	19	1276	30	1431	36
Open heart surgery facilities	469	10	560	12	754	17	795	20
Nuclear mag resonance facility			225	05	837	20	1576	40
Single photon emiss comput tomog					866	20	1386	35
Angioplasty					945	22	940	24

[1] In the 1994 data set there is a service titled 'radiation therapy.' For 1980, 1985 and 1990 data sets, the radiation therapy variable was created using the ratio of the following three services; megavoltage radiation therapy, therapeutic radioisotope facility and x-ray therapy.

25 Hospital Markets with the Highest Market Concentration

Table B1. The 25 hospital markets with the lowest market concentration (1980–1994), using the Hirschman Herfindahl Index (HHI) created with hospital inpatient days

1980		1985	
NAME	**HHI**	**NAME**	**HHI**
Chicago, IL	0.014	Chicago, IL	0.015
Los Angeles-Long Beach, CA	0.016	Los Angeles-Long Beach, CA	0.018
Philadelphia, PA-NJ	0.018	New York, NY	0.019
New York, NY	0.018	Philadelphia, PA-NJ	0.019
Boston, MA-NH	0.023	Boston, MA-NH	0.024
Detroit, MI	0.026	Detroit, MI	0.029
Pittsburgh, PA	0.033	Pittsburgh, PA	0.034
Washington, DC-MD-VA-WV	0.036	Washington, DC-MD-VA-WV	0.036
St. Louis, MO-IL	0.039	Newark, NJ	0.043
Cleveland-Lorain-Elyria, OH	0.039	Oakland, CA	0.043
Newark, NJ	0.041	ST. Louis, MO-IL	0.044
Oakland, CA	0.041	Orange County, CA	0.046
Orange County, CA	0.042	Kansas City, MO-KS	0.048
Atlanta, GA	0.044	Nassau-Suffolk, NY	0.048
Kansas City, MO-KS	0.045	Cleveland-Lorain-Elyria, OH	0.049
Houston, TX	0.046	Atlanta, GA	0.049
Minneapolis-St. Paul, MN-WI	0.048	Houston, TX	0.049
Nassau-Suffolk, NY	0.049	Tampa-St Petersbrg-Clearwter, FL	0.050
Baltimore, MD	0.053	Baltimore, MD	0.052
San Franciso, CA	0.053	San Franciso, CA	0.053
Tampa-St Petersbrg-Clearwter, FL	0.053	San Diego, CA	0.057
Miami, FL	0.054	Riverside-San Bernardino, CA	0.058
San Diego, CA	0.054	Minneapolist-St. Paul, MN-WI	0.058
Milwaukee-Waukesha, WI	0.056	Milwaukee-Waukesha, WI	0.059
Riverside-San Bernardino, CA	0.056	Seattle-Bellevue-Everett, WA	0.063

Table B1. (Continued)

1990		1994	
NAME	**HHI**	**NAME**	**HHI**
Chicago, IL	0.017	Chicago, IL	0.017
Los Angeles-Long Beach, CA	0.018	Los Angeles-Long Beach, CA	0.019
New York, NY	0.019	New York, NY	0.020
Philadelphia, PA-NJ	0.020	Philadelphia, PA-NJ	0.022
Boston, MA-NH	0.026	Boston, MA-NH	0.030
Detroit, MI	0.033	Detroit, MI	0.035
Pittsburgh, PA	0.037	Washington, DC-MD-VA-WV	0.041
Washington, DC-MD-VA-WV	0.038	Pittsburgh, PA	0.045
Orange County, CA	0.044	Orange County, CA	0.046
Newark, NJ	0.046	St. Louis, MO-IL	0.049
St. Louis, MO-IL	0.047	Newark, NJ	0.051
Atlanta, GA	0.048	Kansas City, MO-KS	0.053
Nassau-Suffolk, NY	0.051	Tampa-St Petersbrg-Clearwter,FL	0.054
Oakland, CA	0.052	Riverside-San Bernardino, CA	0.056
Kansas City, MO-KS	0.052	San Diego, CA	0.057
Cleveland-Lorain-Elyria, OH	0.053	Phoenix-Mesa, AZ	0.057
Houston, TX	0.054	Houston, TX	0.058
Tampa-St Petersbrg-Clearwter, FL	0.055	Cleveland-Lorain-Elyria, OH	0.061
Baltimore, MD	0.055	Atlanta, GA	0.061
Riverside-San Bernardino, CA	0.056	Baltimore, MD	0.062
Phoenix-Mesa, AZ	0.059	Oakland, CA	0.062
New Orleans, LA	0.060	Nassau-Suffolk, NY	0.063
San Diego, CA	0.060	New Orleans, LA	0.066
San Francisco, CA	0.066	Minneapolis-St. Paul, MN-WI	0.071
Seattle-Bellevue-Everett, WA	0.067	Dallas, TX	0.072

OLS Regression Results of Efficiency and Community Service Outcomes

Table 19. OLS regression of efficiency outcomes: total expenses per adjusted admission

		1980	1985	1990	1994
	(Constant)	49.36 a	865.62 ***	1386.35 ***	1408.19 ***
		154.18 b	219.51	259.48	293.30
INTERNAL HOSPITAL CHARACTERISTICS					
hospital ownership type (government not-for-profit hospitals is used as the left out category)	private not-for-profit hospital	20.40	−22.30	−47.89	−96.87 *
		23.52	35.23	44.49	49.26
	religious not-for-profit hospital	43.85	59.94	−2.20	−70.34
		32.04	48.03	61.44	68.41
	for-profit hospital	211.18 ***	414.95 ***	527.48 ***	133.06
		34.98	48.63	61.48	70.50
	hospital has a system affiliation	127.53 ***	157.69 ***	110.24 **	66.95
		22.08	28.19	34.83	37.78
hospital size (hospitals with fewer than 100 beds is the left out category)	hospital has 100 to 249 beds	45.78	19.85	125.61 **	104.22 *
		25.18	37.62	47.49	52.00
	hospital has 250 to 399 beds	−18.39	108.73	327.03 ***	335.32 ***
		39.55	56.62	70.67	77.56
	hospital has 400 or more beds	−116.90 *	43.29	394.00 ***	505.40 ***
		52.93	75.02	93.81	102.02

Table 19. (Continued)

		1980	1985	1990	1994
hospital teaching status	hospital is a member of COTH	1142.87 ***	1535.03 ***	2045.09 ***	2521.50 ***
		51.99	68.86	90.61	99.69
	hospital has a medical-school affiliation	356.95 ***	308.49 ***	460.54 ***	651.17 ***
		38.13	51.25	57.81	61.93
	hospital has an intern or residency program	288.38 ***	421.19 ***	561.49 ***	585.34 ***
		41.38	70.87	93.92	85.96
hospital case-mix indicators	proportion of operations that are inpatient operations	−41.92	−21.05	213.20	622.38 ***
		57.02	87.43	116.87	134.10
	Medicaid ip days as a proportion of adj ip days	1985.85 ***	595.03 **	471.00	1665.44 ***
		189.03	205.49	241.65	238.37
	Medicare ip days as a proportion of adj ip days	1507.86 ***	1408.96 ***	2189.71 ***	2240.92 ***
		95.89	141.86	176.21	189.63
other internal hospital characteristics	ratio of full-time LPNs to full-time RNs	−502.50 ***	−782.64 ***	−1097.28 ***	−1021.63 ***
		66.13	107.57	138.65	164.95

Table 19. (Continued)

	1980	1985	1990	1994
average length of stay using ipdays	137.09 ***	101.84 ***	96.25 ***	82.66 ***
	3.65	3.93	3.37	3.08
ratio of technology services	825.69 ***	1067.37 ***	963.60 ***	1091.24 ***
	53.69	82.51	96.22	100.73

HOSPITAL ENVIRONMENTAL CHARACTERISTICS

	1980	1985	1990	1994
ratio of specialists to patient-care MDs	148.11	118.04	227.23	–125.23
5-yr chng in MD ratio	151.78	213.63	253.15	258.32
	281.35	–73.31	–530.35	–43.75
	193.20	246.58	319.08	342.57
proportion of population age 65 and over	–1325.96 ***	–1819.14 ***	–3215.52 ***	–4230.07 ***
5-yr chng in the proportion of population age 65+	379.17	539.11	640.40	689.47
	747.82	–2595.45	1829.98	1352.74
per capita income – 1994 dollars	1379.88	1973.38	2446.31	3933.90
	0.05 ***	0.07 ***	0.08 ***	0.09 ***
	0.01	0.01	0.01	0.01

NOTE: The state location of the hospital is controlled for with the use of dummy variables. New York State is used as the left out category.

Table 19. (Continued)

	1980	1985	1990	1994
5-yr chng in the per capita income	-147.02	-466.40 **	-215.47	-189.72
unemployment rate	138.51	165.55	311.17	335.18
	2.64	21.53 **	32.90 **	35.96 **
	5.10	6.71	11.85	12.11
proportion of population who are HMO members	594.90 ***	983.42 ***	-5.25	-601.09 ***
Herfindahl index using inpatient days	127.93	157.97	173.02	177.60
	-108.94 **	-163.65 *	-292.38 ***	-243.66 *
	41.73	63.60	80.66	94.92
hospital located in rural area	-188.14 ***	-278.70 ***	-318.13 ***	-213.80 **
	28.80	45.66	58.53	72.40
R^2	0.71	0.66	0.66	0.67
N	4558.00	4502.00	4314.00	3956.00

$*p < .05, **p < .01, ***p < .001$
a - unstandardized regression coefficient
b - standardized error

Table 20. OLS regression of efficiency outcomes: full-time equivalent employees per adjusted census

		1980	1985	1990	1994
	(Constant)	3.935 ***	4.480 ***	4.877 ***	4.980 ***
		0.154	0.192	0.218	0.306
INTERNAL HOSPITAL CHARACTERISTICS					
hospital ownership type (government not-for-profit hospitals is used as the left out category)	private not-for-profit hospital	−0.056 *	−0.121 ***	−0.173 ****	−0.202 ****
		0.023	0.031	0.037	0.051
	religious not-for-profit hospital	−0.004	−0.080	−0.154 **	−0.262 ***
		0.032	0.042	0.052	0.071
	for-profit hospital	−0.224 ***	−0.289 ***	−0.335 ****	−0.310 ****
		0.035	0.042	0.052	0.074
	hospital has a system affiliation	−0.023	−0.082 ***	−0.163 ****	−0.151 ***
		0.022	0.025	0.029	0.039
hospital size (hospitals with fewer than 100 beds is the left out category)	hospital has 100 to 249 beds	−0.127 ***	−0.330 ***	−0.357 ***	−0.475 ***
		0.025	0.033	0.040	0.054
	hospital has 250 to 399 beds	−0.178 ***	−0.311 ***	−0.340 ***	−0.512 ***
		0.040	0.049	0.059	0.081
	hospital has 400 or more beds	−0.198 ***	−0.317 ***	−0.325 ***	−0.423 ***
		0.053	0.065	0.079	0.107
hospital teaching status	hospital is a member of COTH	0.882 ***	1.066 ***	1.229 ***	1.487 ***
		0.052	0.060	0.076	0.104

Table 20. (Continued)

	1980	1985	1990	1994
hospital has a medical-school affiliation	0.290 ***	0.273 ***	0.294 ***	0.496 ***
	0.038	0.045	0.049	0.065
hospital has an intern or residency program	0.166 ***	0.282 ***	0.232 **	0.289 **
	0.041	0.062	0.079	0.090
hospital case-mix indicators				
proportion of operations that are inpatient operations	-0.077	0.149	0.397 ***	0.205
	0.057	0.076	0.098	0.140
Medicaid ip days as a proportion of adj ip days	0.876 ***	-0.187	-0.914 ***	-1.055 ***
	0.189	0.179	0.203	0.249
Medicare ip days as a proportion of adj ip days	0.706 ***	0.509 ***	0.587 ***	1.228 ***
	0.096	0.124	0.148	0.198
other internal hospital characteristics				
ratio of full-time LPNs to full-time RNs	-0.188 **	-0.305 **	-0.231 *	-0.276
	0.066	0.094	0.116	0.172
average length of stay using ipdays	-0.118 ***	-0.135 ***	-0.109 ***	-0.110 ***
	0.004	0.003	0.003	0.003

Table 20. (Continued)

	1980	1985	1990	1994
HOSPITAL ENVIRONMENTAL CHARACTERISTICS				
ratio of technology services	0.401 ***	0.379 ***	0.407 ***	0.333 **
	0.054	0.072	0.081	0.105
ratio of specialists to patient-care MDs	-0.05	-0.52 **	-0.31	-0.35
	0.15	0.19	0.21	0.27
5-yr chng in MD ratio	0.18	0.15	0.23	-0.08
	0.19	0.22	0.27	0.36
proportion of population age 65 and over	-1.89 ***	-1.45 **	-2.27 ***	-2.31 **
	0.38	0.47	0.54	0.72
5-yr chng in the proportion of population age 65+	2.71 *	6.89 ***	1.64	7.23
	1.38	1.72	2.05	4.11
per capita income-1994 dollars	1.70E-06	1.22E-05 *	6.00E-07	1.11E-05
	5.18E-06	6.17E-06	6.25E-06	8.51E-06
5-yr chng in the per capita income	-0.09	-0.34 *	-0.10	-0.25
	0.14	0.14	0.26	0.35

NOTE: The state location of the hospital is controlled for with the use of dummy variables. New York State is used as the left out category.

Table 20. (Continued)

	1980	1985	1990	1994
unemployment rate	-0.01 **	-0.01	-0.02 *	-0.03 **
	0.01	0.01	0.01	0.01
proportion of population who are HMO members	-0.12	0.18	-0.28	-0.33
	0.13	0.14	0.15	0.19
Herfindahl index using inpatient days	-0.05	-0.07	-0.03	0.03
	0.04	0.06	0.07	0.10
hospital located in rural area	-0.04	-0.03	-0.17 ***	-0.22 **
	0.03	0.04	0.05	0.08
R^2	0.43	0.49	0.54	0.53
N	4558	4502	4314	3956

*p < .05, ** p < .01, *** p < .001
a - unstandardized regression coefficient
b - standardized error

Table 21. OLS regression of community-service outcomes: ratio of emergency room visits per adjusted inpatient day

	1980	1985	1990	1994
(Constant)	0.61 ****	0.60 ****	0.69 ****	0.68 ****
	0.04	0.04	0.04	0.05
INTERNAL HOSPITAL CHARACTERISTICS				
hospital ownership type (government not-for-profit hospitals is used as the left out category)				
private not-for-profit hospital	-0.04 ***	-0.04***	-0.03***	-0.03 ***
	0.01	0.01	0.01	0.01
religious not-for-profit hospital	-0.05***	-0.06 ***	-0.04 ***	-0.06 ***
	0.01	0.01	0.01	0.01
for-profit hospital	-0.09 ***	-0.10 ***	-0.07 ***	-0.08 ***
	0.01	0.01	0.01	0.01
hospital has a system affiliation	0.02 ***	0.02 ***	0.02 ***	0.02 ***
	0.01	0.01	0.01	0.01
hospital size (hospitals with fewer than 100 beds is the left out category)				
hospital has 100 to 249 beds	-0.01	-0.05 ***	-0.09 ***	-0.12 ***
	0.01	0.01	0.01	0.01
hospital has 250 to 399 beds	-0.03 ***	-0.09 ***	-0.16 ***	-0.21 ***
	0.01	0.01	0.01	0.01
hospital has 400 or more beds	-0.06 ***	-0.12 ***	-0.19 ***	-0.26 ***
	0.01	0.01	0.01	0.02

Table 21. (Continued)

	1980	1985	1990	1994
hospital teaching status				
hospital is a member of COTH	-0.02	-8.89E-04	-0.02	-0.03
	0.01	0.01	0.01	0.02
hospital has a medical-school affiliation	-2.04E-03	-0.01	-0.02	-0.01
hospital has an intern or residency program	0.01	0.01	0.01	0.01
	-0.02 *	-0.02	-0.02	-0.01
hospital case-mix indicators				
proportion of operations that are inpatient operations	0.01	0.01	0.01	0.01
	-0.01	-0.03	-0.02	-0.02
Medicaid ip days as a proportion of adj ip days	0.01	0.02	0.02	0.02
	-0.12 **	-0.01	-0.07	-0.13 **
Medicare ip days as a proportion of adj ip days	0.04	0.04	0.04	0.04
	-0.20 ***	-0.10 ***	-0.04	0.04
other internal hospital characteristics				
ratio of full-time LPNs to full-time RNs	0.02	0.03	0.03	0.03
	1.25E-03	-0.02	-0.04 *	-0.04
	0.02	0.02	0.02	0.03

Table 21. (Continued)

	1980	1985	1990	1994
average length of stay using ipdays	−0.02 ***	−0.02 ***	−0.01 ***	−0.01 ***
ratio of technology services	8.33E-04	7.01E-04	5.38E-04	5.37E-04
	−0.02	−0.07 ***	−0.05 ***	−0.04 *
	0.01	0.01	0.02	0.02

HOSPITAL ENVIRONMENTAL CHARACTERISTICS

	1980	1985	1990	1994
ratio of specialists to patient-care MDs	0.03	0.04	0.09 *	0.09 *
	0.03	0.04	0.04	0.05
5-yr chng in MD ratio	−0.01	1.61E-04	−0.05	0.08
	0.04	0.04	0.05	0.06
proportion of population age 65 and over	−0.19 *	−0.60 ***	−0.85 ***	−0.94 ***
	0.09	0.10	0.10	0.12
5-yr chng in the proportion of population age 65+	−0.50	1.21 ***	0.28	−0.49
	0.31	0.35	0.39	0.69
per capita income-1994 dollars	4.00E-07	1.75E-06	7.62E-09	−1.97E-08
	1.18E-06	1.26E-06	1.19E-06	1.42E-06

NOTE: The state location of the hospital is controlled for with the use of dummy variables. New York State is used as the left out category.

Table 21. (Continued)

	1980	1985	1990	1994
5-yr chng in the per capita income	0.05	0.05	−0.14 **	0.08
	0.03	0.03	0.05	0.06
unemployment rate	3.25E-03 **	4.89E-03 ***	7.91E-03 ***	6.14E-03 **
	1.16E-03	1.20E-03	1.89E-03	2.11E-03
proportion of population who are HMO members	−0.04	0.01	−0.05	−0.07 *
	0.03	0.03	0.03	0.03
Herfindahl index using inpatient days	0.02	0.02 *	0.02	0.04 *
	0.01	0.01	0.01	0.02
hospital located in rural area	−0.01	−0.01	−0.01	−0.04 ***
	0.01	0.01	0.01	0.01
R^2	0.32	0.36	0.43	0.44
N	4558	4502	4314	3956

*$p < .05$, **$p < .01$, ***$p < .001$
a - unstandardized regression coefficient
b - standardized error

Table 22. OLS regression of community-service outcomes: ratio of outpatient visits per adjusted inpatient day

	1980	1985	1990	1994
(Constant)	0.310 *** a	0.373 ***	0.571 ***	0.701 ***
	0.011 b	0.012	0.014	0.018
INTERNAL HOSPITAL CHARACTERISTICS				
hospital ownership type (government not-for-profit hospitals is used as the left out category)				
private not-for-profit hospital	-0.009 ***	-0.005 **	-0.006 *	-0.005
	0.002	0.002	0.002	0.003
religious not-for-profit hospital	-0.013 ***	-0.009 ***	-0.010**	-0.004
	0.002	0.003	0.003	0.004
for-profit hospital	-0.037 ***	-0.031 ***	-0.040 ***	-0.039 ***
	0.003	0.003	0.003	0.004
hospital has a system affiliation	0.006 ***	0.001	0.002	-0.001
	0.002	0.001	0.002	0.002
hospital size (hospitals with fewer than 100 beds is the left out category)				
hospital has 100 to 249 beds	-0.012 ***	-0.014 ***	-0.029***	-0.033 ***
	0.002	0.002	0.003	0.003
hospital has 250 to 399 beds	-0.019 ***	-0.034***	-0.059 ***	-0.064 ***
	0.003	0.003	0.004	0.005
hospital has 400 or more beds	-0.025 ***	-0.043 ***	-0.074 ***	-0.077 ***
	0.004	0.004	0.005	0.006
hospital teaching status hospital is a member of COTH	0.018 ***	-0.005	-0.019 ***	-0.042 ***
	0.004	0.004	0.005	0.006

Table 22. (Continued)

	1980	1985	1990	1994
hospital has a medical-school affiliation	0.006 *	−0.006 *	−0.010 **	−0.015***
	0.003	0.003	0.003	0.004
hospital has an intern or residency program	−0.005	−0.014 ***	−0.015 **	−0.018 ***
	0.003	0.004	0.005	0.005
hospital case-mix indicators proportion of operations that are inpatient operations	−0.039 ***	−0.066 **	−0.093 ***	−0.119 ***
	0.004	0.005	0.006	0.008
Medicaid ip days as a proportion of adj ip days	−0.099 ***	−0.084 ***	−0.179 ***	−0.349 ***
	0.014	0.011	0.013	0.014
Medicare ip days as a proportion of adj ip days	−0.166 ***	−0.172 ***	−0.276 ***	−0.436 ***
	0.007	0.007	0.009	0.012
other internal hospital characteristics ratio of full-time Lens to full-time RNs	−0.008	0.005	−0.007	0.019
	0.005	0.006	0.007	0.010
average length of stay using ipdays	−0.004 ***	−0.003 ***	−0.003 ***	−0.003 ***
	0.000	0.000	0.000	0.000

Table 22. (Continued)

	1980	1985	1990	1994
ratio of technology services	-0.007	-0.012 **	-0.032 ***	-0.027 ***
	0.004	0.004	0.005	0.006
HOSPITAL ENVIRONMENTAL CHARACTERISTICS				
ratio of specialists to patient-care MDs	0.010	-0.003	-0.008	-0.013
	0.011	0.011	0.014	0.016
5-yr chng in MD ratio	-0.008	0.005	0.017	-0.014
	0.014	0.013	0.017	0.021
proportion of population age 65 and over	0.049	0.003	-0.002	0.019
	0.027	0.028	0.034	0.042
5-yr chng in the proportion of population age 65+	-0.129	-0.016	0.273 *	-0.328
	0.100	0.104	0.131	0.239
per capita income- 1994 dollars	-7.629E-07 *	-5.975E-07	-1.831E-06 ***	-2.102E-06 ***
	3.761E-07	3.716E-07	3.979E-07	4.956E-07
5-yr chng in the per capita income	0.001	0.023 **	-0.033 *	0.014
	0.010	0.009	0.017	0.020
unemployment rate	0.001 **	0.001 *	3.714E-04	0.001

NOTE: The state location of the hospital is controlled for with the use of dummy variables. New York State is used as the left out category.

Table 22. (Continued)

	1980	1985	1990	1994
proportion of population who are HMO members	3.699E-04 0.007	3.530E-04 −0.018 *	0.001 −0.026 **	0.001 −0.026 *
Herfindahl index using inpatient days	0.009 −0.001	0.008 0.001	0.009 0.006	0.011 0.013 *
hospital located in rural area	0.003 0.001 0.002	0.003 0.002 0.002	0.004 0.005 0.003	0.006 0.004 0.004
R^2	0.394	0.433	0.605	0.680
N	4558	4502	4314	3956

*p < .05, ** p < .01, *** p < .001

a - unstandardized regression coefficient

b - standardized error

Table 23. T-test Results Comparing Hospital-Ownership Regression Coefficients

Year	Hospital Outcome	Comparison I for profit/ private not-for-profit	Comparison II for profit/ religious not-for-profit	Comparison III private not-for-profit/ religious not-for-profit
1980	Expenses per adjusted admission	6.38 **	4.70 **	0.81
	Full time equivalents per adjusted dailycensus	6.60 **	6.93 **	1.91
	Emergency room visits per adjusted inpatient day	8.79 **	5.65 **	2.22 *
	Outpatient visits per adjusted inpatient day	12.74 **	8.97 **	2.17 *
1985	Expenses per adjusted admission	11.18 **	7.58 **	1.92
	Full time equivalents per adjusted dailycensus	5.70 **	5.56 **	1.18
	Emergency room visits per adjusted inpatient day	7.72 **	4.06 **	2.82 **
	Outpatient visits per adjusted inpatient day	12.30 **	8.45 **	1.97 *

Table 23. (Continued)

Year	Hospital Outcome	Comparison I for profit/ private not-for-profit	Comparison II for profit/ religious not-for-profit	Comparison III private not-for-profit/ religious not-for-profit
1990	Expenses per adjusted admission	11.78 **	8.78 **	0.85
	Full time equivalents per adjusted dailycensus	5.53 **	4.79 **	0.45
	Emergency room visits per adjusted inpatient day	6.50 **	3.93 **	1.62
	Outpatient visits per adjusted inpatient day	10.67 **	7.30 **	1.60
1994	Expenses per adjusted admission	3.80 **	2.83 **	0.29
	Full time equivalents per adjusted dailycensus	3.12 **	1.50	1.30
	Emergency room visits per adjusted inpatient day	4.80 **	2.24 *	2.11 *
	Outpatient visits per adjusted inpatient day	6.69 **	5.89 **	0.68

significance levels: * p < .05, ** p < .01

References

Abbas, F. M., Sert, M. B. Rosenshein, N. B., Zahyrak, M. L., and J. L. Currie. 1997. "Prolonged Stays of OB/GYN Patients in the Surgical Intensive Care Unit." *Journal of Reproductive Medicine* 42:179–183.

Abraham, L. K. 1993. *Mama Might Be Better Off Dead: The Failure of Health Care in America.* Chicago: The University of Chicago Press.

Albrecht, G. L., Slobodkin, D., and R. J. Rydman. 1996. "The Role of Emergency Departments in American Health Care." In *Research in the Sociology of Health Care,* ed. J. J. Kronenfeld, 289–318. Greenwich, CT: JAI Press.

Alexander, J. A., Kaluzny, A. S. and S. C. Middleton. 1986. "Organizational Growth, Survival and Death in the U.S. Hospital Industry: A Population Ecology Perspective." *Social Science and Medicine* 22:303–308.

Altman, S. H. and D. Shactman. 1997. "Why should we worry about hospitals' high administrative costs?" *The New England Journal of Medicine.* 336:798–99.

Altman, S. H., and D. A. Young. 1993. "A Decade of Medicare's Prospective Payment System—Success or Failure?" *Journal of American Health Policy.* March/April: 11–19.

American Hospital Association. 1995. *The AHA Profile of Hospital Statistics.* Chicago: American Hospital Association.

American Hospital Association. 1993/94. *The AHA Profile of Hospital Statistics.* Chicago: American Hospital Association.

American Hospital Association. 1994. *1994 AHA Guide.* Chicago: American Hospital Association.

American Hospital Association. 1992. *1992 AHA Guide.* Chicago: American Hospital Association.

Anderson, G. F., and L. T. Kohn. 1996. "Hospital Employment Trends in California, 1982–1994." *Health Affairs* 15(1):152–158.

Andrulis, D., Kellerman A., Hintz E., Hackman, B., and V. Weslowski. 1991. "Emergency Departments and Crowding in U.S. Teaching Hospitals." *Annals of Emergency Medicine* 20:980–986.

Archer, B., 1991. "To the Editor." *The New England Journal of Medicine* 325:1316.

Arrington, B. and C. C. Haddock. 1990. "Who Really Profits from Not-For-Profits?" *Health Services Research* 25:291–304.

Baker, D. W., Stevens, C. and R. H. Brook. 1995. "Determinants of Emergency Department Use by Ambulatory Patients at an Urban Public Hospital." *Annals of Emergency Medicine.* 25:311–316.

Baker, L. C., and L. S. Baker. 1994. "Excess Cost of Emergency Department Visits for Nonurgent Care." *Health Affairs* (Winter):163–171.

Baron, J. N., Dobbin, F. R. and P. D. Jennings. 1986. "War and Peace: The Evolution of Modern Personnel Administration in U.S. Industry." *American Journal of Sociology* 92:350–383.

Barrett, M. W. 1995. "Downsizing: Doing it Rationally." *Nursing Management* 26:24–29.

Bazzoli, G. J. and E. J. Mackenzie. 1995. "Trauma Centers in the United States: Identification and Examination of Key Characteristics." *Journal of Trauma* 38:103–110.

Becker, E. R. and F. Sloan. 1985. "Hospital Ownership and Performance." *Economic Inquiry* 23:21–35.

Becker, E. R. and B. Steinwald. 1981. "Determinants of Hospital Casemix Complexity." *Health Services Research* 16:439–458.

Binder, A. B. 1993. *Finding and Using Economic Information: A Guide to Sources and Interpretation.* California: Bristlecone Books.

Blaisdell, F. W. 1994. "Development of the City-County (Public Hospital)." *Arch Surg* 129:760–764.

Blewett, L. A., Kane, R. L. and M. Finch. 1995/1996. "Hospital Ownership of Post-Acute Care: Does it increase Access to Post-Acute Care Services." *Inquiry* 32:457–67.

Braveman, P., Kessel, W., Egerter, S. and J. Richmond. 1997. "Early Discharge and Evidence-based Practice: Good Science and Good Judgement." *Journal of the American Medical Association,* 278:334–336.

Brier, P. 1997. "At Risk: Health Care for the Poor." *New York Times.* (January 18):21.

Brown, E. 1983. "Public Hospitals on the Brink: Their Problems and Their Options." *Journal of Health Politics, Policy and Law* 7(Winter):927–44.

Bureau of Health Professions. 1997. *User Documentation for the Area Resource File (ARF).* Office of Research and Planning: Department of Health and Human Services.

Burns, Lawton R. 1990. "The Transformation of the American Hospital: From Community Institution toward Business Enterprise." *Comparative Social Research* 12:77–112.

Burstin, H. R., Lipsitz, S. R., Udvarhelyi, S. and T. A. Brennan. 1993. "The Effect of Hospital Financial Characteristics on Quality of Care." *Journal of the American Medical Association* 270:845–849.

Cerne, F. 1995. "Street Wise: Analysts upbeat about providers' response to volatile market." *Hospitals & Health Networks:* 38–45.

Chang and Tuckman. 1988. "The Profits of Not-For-Profit Hospitals," *Journal of Health Politics, Policy and Law* 13:547–64.

Classen, D. C., Pestotnik, S. L., Scott, E. R., Lloyed, J. F. and J. P. Burke. 1997. "Adverse Drug Events in Hospitalized Patients: Excess Length of Stay, Extra Costs and Attributable Mortality." *Journal of the American Medical Association* 277:301–306.

Cleverly, W. O. 1992a. "Financial and Operating Performance of Systems: Voluntary versus investor-owned." *Topics in Health Care Financing* 18:63–73.

———. 1992b. *Essentials of Health Care Finance.* Gaithersburg, Maryland: Aspen Publishers.

Coddington, D., Palmquist, L., and W. Trollinger. 1985. "Strategies for Survival in the Hospital Industry." *Harvard Business Review* (May–June):129–38.

Cohen, J. and P. Cohen. 1983. *Applied Multiple Regression/Correlation Analysis for the Behavioral Sciences.* London: Lawrence Erlbaum Associates.

Committee on Implications of For-Profit Enterprise in Health Care. 1986. "Access to Care." In *For-Profit Enterprise in Health Care.* ed. D. H. Gray, 97–126. Washington, DC: National Academy Press.

Consumer Reports Editors. 1996. "Can HMOs Help Solve the Health Care Crisis?" *Consumer Reports* (October):28–33.

Coyne, J. S. 1982. "Hospital Performance in Multihospital Systems: A Comparative Study of System and Independent Hospitals." *Health Services Research* 17:303–329.

Culler, S. D., Holmes, A. M. and B. Gutierrez. 1995. "Expected Hospital Costs of Knee Replacement for Rural Residents by Location of Service." *Medical Care* 33:1188–209.

Custer, W. S. and R. J. Wilke. 1991. "Teaching hospital costs: the effect of medical staff characteristics." *Health Services Research* 25:831–857.

DiMaggio, P. J. 1991. "Constructing an Organizational Field as a Professional Project." In *The New Institutionalism in Organizational Analysis,* eds. W. W. Powell and P. J. DiMaggio, 267–292. Chicago: The University of Chicago Press.

DiMaggio, P. J. 1986. "Support for the Arts from Private Foundations. in *Nonprofit Enterprise in the Arts*, ed. P. J. DiMaggio, 113–39. New York: Oxford University Press.

DiMaggio, P. J. and W. W. Powell. 1983. "The Iron Cage Revisited: Institutional Isomorphism and Collective Rationality in Organizational Fields." *American Sociological Review* 48:147–60.

Dobbin, F. and T. J. Dowd. 1997. "How Policy Shapes Competition: Early Railroad Foundings in Massachusetts." *Administrative Science Quarterly* 42:501–529.

Dobbin, F., Sutton J. R., Meyer J. W. and W. R. Scott. 1993. "Equal Opportunity and the Construction of Internal Labor Markets." *American Journal of Sociology* 99:396–427.

Dowd, T. J. and F. Dobbin. 1998. "Was There a Market Before Antitrust?: Public Policy and Railroad Strategy in Early America." in *Constructing Markets and Industries*, ed. J. Porac and M. Ventresa, Forthcoming. New York: Pergamon Press.

Duffy, Sarah Q. and Dean E. Farley. 1995. "Patterns of Decline among Inpatient Procedures." *Public Health Reports* 110:674–681.

Engelman, R. M. 1996. "Mechanisms to Reduce Hospital Stays." *Annals of Thoracic Surgery* 61:S26–S29.

Estes, C. L. and J. H. Swan. 1994. "Privatization, System Membership and Access to Home Health Care for the Elderly." *Milbank Quarterly* 72:277–298.

Fennel, M. L. and J. A. Alexander. 1993. "Perspectives on Organizational Change in the US Medical Sector." *Annual Review of Sociology* 19:89–112.

Fennel, Mary L. and Jeffrey A. Alexander. 1987. "The Effects of Environmental Characteristics on the Structure of Hospital Clusters." *Administrative Science Quarterly* 25:485–510.

Finkler, S. A. 1982. "The Distinction Between Cost and Charges." *Annals of Internal Medicine* 96:102–109.

Fligstein, N. 1991. "The Structural Transformation of American Industry: An Institutional Account of the Causes of Diversification in the Largest Firms, 1919–1979." In *The New Institutionalism in Organizational Analysis*, ed. W.W. Powell and P.J. DiMaggio, 311–336. Chicago: The University of Chicago Press.

Fligstein, N. 1987. "The Intraorganizational Power Struggle: Rise of Finance Personnel to Top Leadership in Large Corporations, 1919–1979." *American Sociological Review* 52:44–58.

Fligstein, N. 1985. "The Spread of the Multidivsional Firm, 1919–79." *American Sociological Review* 50:377–391.

Fox, D. M. and D. C. Schaffer. 1991. "Tax Administration as Health Policy: Hospitals, the Internal Revenue Service and the Courts." *Journal of Health Politics, Policy and Law* 16:251–279.

Frank, R. G. and D. S. Salkever. 1991. "The Supply of Charity Services Provided by Nonprofit Hospitals: Motives and Market Structures." *RAND Journal of Economics* 22:430–445.

Friedman, B. and D. Farley. 1995. "Strategic Responses by Hospitals to Increased Financial Risk in the 1980s." *Health Services Research* 30: 467–488.

Friedman, L. H. and J. Jorgensen. 1994. "Physician's Influence on the Decision to Acquire Magnetic Resonance Imagers in Acute Care Hospitals." *International Journal of Technology Assessment in Health Care* 10:667–674.

Frist, T. and J. Campbell. 1981. "Outlook for Hospitals: Systems are the Solution." *Harvard Business Review* (September–October):132.

General Accounting Office. 1993. *Report to the chairman, Subcommittee on Health for Families and the Uninsured, Committee on Finance, U.S. Senate: emergency departments unevenly affected by growth and change in patient use.* Washington D.C.: Government Printing Office, (Publication no. GAO/HRD-93-4.)

General Accounting Office. 1989. *Medicare: Indirect Medical Payments are Too High.* Washington, D.C.: Government Printing Office, Publication GAO/HRD-89-33.

Ginzberg, E. 1988. "For-Profit Medicine: A Reassessment. *New England Journal of Medicine* 319:757–61.

Goldsmith, J. 1981. *Can Hospital's Survive?* Irwin Professional Publishers.

Goodwin, E. J. et al. 1989. "Access to Health Care: Medicare and the Poor Elderly," In *Poverty and Health in the United States*, ed. M. I. Krasner. New York: United Hospital Fund.

Grannemann, T. W., Brown, R. S., and M. V. Pauly. 1986. "Estimating Hospital Costs: A Multiple-Output Analysis." *Journal of Health Economics* 5:107–127.

Gray, B. 1993. "Ownership Matters: Health Reform and the Future of Nonprofit Healthcare." *Inquiry* 30:352–361.

Gray, B. H. 1991. *The Profit Motive and Patient Care: The Changing Accountability of Doctors and Hospitals.* Cambridge, Massachusetts: Harvard University Press.

Greene, J. 1995. "A delicate balancing act." *Modern Healthcare* 25:34–40.

Grumbach, K., Keane, D., and A. Bindman. 1993. "Primary Care and Public Emergency Department Overcrowding." *American Journal of Public Health* 83:372–378.

Guterman, S., Ashby, J. and T. Greene. 1996. "Hospital Cost Growth Down: Unprecedented Cost Constraint by Hospitals has Maintained their Bottom Line. But Can it Continue?" *Health Affairs* 15:134–139.

Hadley, J., and K. Swartz. 1989. "The Impact of Hospital Costs Between 1980 and 1984 of Hospital Rate Regulation, Competition, and Changes in Health Insurance Coverage." *Inquiry* 26:35–47.

Hannan, E. L., Siu, A. L., Kumar, D., Kilburn, H., and M. R. Chassin. 1995. "The Decline in Coronary Artery Bypass Graft Surgery Mortality in New York State." *Journal of the American Medical Association* 273: 209–213.

Hannan, M. T. and J. H. Freeman. 1977. "The Population Ecology of Organizations. *American Journal of Sociology* 82:929–64.

Hansman, Henry. 1980. "The Role of Nonprofit Enterprise." *Yale Law Journal* 89:835–901.

Hardy, M. 1993. *Regression with Dummy Variables.* Sage University Paper series on Quantitative Applications in the Social Sciences, 07-093. Newbury Park, CA: Sage.

Hartz, A. J., Krakauer, H., Kuhn, E. M., Young, M., S. J. Jacobsen, Greer, G., Muenz, L., Katzoff, M., Bailey, R. C. and A. A. Rimm. 1989. "Hospital Characteristics and Mortality Rates." *The New England Journal of Medicine.* 321:1720–1725.

Herzlinger, R. E., and W. S. Krasker. 1987. "Who Profits from Nonprofits?" *Harvard Business Review* 93–105.

Homer, C .G., Bradham, D. D., and M. Rushefsky. 1984. "To the Editor, Investor-Owned and Not-For-Profit Hospitals: Beyond the Cost and Revenue Debate." *Health Affairs:* 133–136.

Hospitals & Health Networks. 1996. "Human Resources." *Hospitals & Health Networks,* October 20:11.

Hospitals & Health Networks. 1995. "Heavy Managed Care Means Slower Rise in Hospital Costs." *Hospitals & Health Networks* 14:1996.

Hultman, Cheryl I. 1991. "Uncompensated Care before and after Prospective Payment: The Role of Hospital Location and Ownership." *Health Services Research* 26:614–22.

Jaffe, Greg and Monica Langley. 1996. "Generous to a Fault? Fledgling Charities Get Billions from the Sales of Nonprofit Hospitals." *Wall Street Journal* (November 6):A1.

Jee, M. 1993. "Texas Links Charity Care, Hospital Tax-Exempt Status." *Journal of American Health Policy* 3.

Johannes, Laura. 1996. "More HMOs Order Outpatient Mastectomies." *Wall Street Journal* (November 6):B1.

Johantgen, Mary E., Coffey, Rosanna M.. Harris, D. Robert, Levy, H., and J. J. Clinton. 1995. "Treating Early-Stage Breast Cancer: Hospital Characteristics Associated with Breast Conserving Surgery." *American Journal of Public Health* 85:1432–34.

Kahn, R. M. 1996. "The Ritziest Hospitals in Town." *Boston Magazine* 88:68–73, 115–120.

Kane, Nancy. 1993. "Report on the Financial Resources of Major Hospitals in Boston." Department of Health and Hospitals: Boston.

Kellerman, A. L. 1994. "Nonurgent Emergency Department Visits: Meeting an Unmet Need." *Journal of the American Medical Association* 271: 1953–1954.

Kendall, D. 1998. *Social Problems in a Diverse Society.* London. Allyn and Bacon.

Knoke, D. and G. W. Bohrnstedt. 1994. *Statistics for Social Data Analysis.* Itasca, Illinois: F.E. Peacock Publishers, Inc.

Kuhn, E. M., Hartz, A. J., Gottlieb, M.S., and A. A. Rimm. 1991. "The Relationship of Hospital Characteristics and the Results of Peer Review in Six Large States." *Medical Care* 29:1028–1038.

Kuttner, R. 1996. "Columbia/HCA and the Resurgence of the For-Profit Hospital Business." *New England Journal of Medicine* 335:446–51.

Laumann. Edward O., Galaskiewicz, Joseph. and Peter Marsden. 1978. "Community Structure as Interorganizational Linkage." *Annual Review of Sociology* 4:455–84.

Lawrence, Paul R. and Jay W. Lorsch. 1967. *Organization and Environment.* Cambridge, Massachusetts: Harvard University Press.

Levit, B. and C. Nass. 1989. "The Lid on the Garbage Can: Institutional Constraints on Decision Making in the Technical Core of College-Text Publishers." *Administrative Science Quarterly* 34:190–207.

Lumsdon, K., 1994. "Ready for Cost Cutting? One Hospital Mobilizes its Resources." *Hospital & Health Networks. 68(23):* 62.

Lutz, Sandy. 1994. "Not-For-Profits up for Grabs by the Giants: Teaching, Church-Affiliated Hospitals Ponder Deals with Investor-Owned Firms." *Modern Healthcare:* 24–30.

Mann, J., Melnick, G., Bamezai, A., and J. Zwanziger. 1995. "Uncompensated Care: Hospitals' Responses to Fiscal Pressures." *Health Affairs* 236–270.

Mantil, J., R. Willett, and W. Sawyer. 1991. "Medical High-Technology Assessment and Implementation in A Community Hospital: Nuclear Magnetic Resonance." *Biomedical Instrumentation & Technology* 25: 289–296.

Marmor, Theodore R., Schlesinger, Mark and Richard W. Smithey. 1987. "Nonprofit Organizations and Health Care." In *The Nonprofit Sector: A Research Handbook,* ed. W.W. Powell, 221–240. New Haven, CT: Yale University Press.

McNamara, P., Witte, R. and A. Koning. 1993. "Patchwork Access: Primary Care in EDs on the rise." *Hospitals:* 44–46.

Menke, T. J. 1997. "The Effect of Chain Membership on Hospital Costs." *Health Services Research* 32:177–196.

Messinger, Sheldon L. 1955. "Organizational Transformation: A Case Study of Declining Social Movement." *American Sociological Review* 20:3–10.

Meyer, John W. and Richard W. Scott. 1983. *Organizational Environments: Ritual and Rationality.* Beverly Hills, California: Sage.

Meyer, John W. and Brian Rowan. 1977. "Institutionalized Organizations: Formal Structure as Myth and Ceremony." *American Journal of Sociology* 83:364–385.

Mitchell W. 1995. "Medical Diagnostic Imaging Manufacturers." In *Organizations in Industry: Strategy, Structure, and Selection* ed. G. R. Carroll and M. T. Hannan, 244–272. New York: Oxford University Press.

Moore, C. M., Ahmed, I., Mouallem, R., May, W., Ehlayel, M., and R. U. Sorensen. 1997. "Care of Asthma: Allergy Clinic Versus Emergency Room." *Annals of Allergy, Asthma and Immunology* 78:373–380.

Morey, R., Ozcan, Y., Retzlaff-Roberts, D., and D. Fine. 1995. "Estimating the Hospital-Wide Cost Differentials Warranted for Teaching Hospitals." *Medical Care* 33: 531–532.

Morrisey, M. A., Wedig, G. J. and M. Hassan. 1996 "Do Nonprofit Hospital Pay Their Way?" *Health Affairs* 15:132–144.

Neter, John, Wasserman, William and Michael H. Kutner. 1990. *Applied Linear Statistical Models.* Homewood, IL: Irwin.

Newhouse, J. P. 1993. "An Iconoclastic View of Health Cost Containment." *Health Affairs* 12:152.

Norton, E. C. and D. O. Staiger. 1994. "How Hospitals Ownership Affects Access to Care for the Uninsured." *Rand Journal of Economics* 25:171–85.

O'Donnel, J. W. and J. H. Taylor. 1990. "The Bounds of Charity; the Current Status of the Hospital Property-Tax exemption." *The New England Journal of Medicine* 322: 65–67.

Orr, S. T., Charney, E., Strauss, J., and B. Bloom. 1991. "Emergency Room Use by Low Income Children with a Regular Source of Health Care." *Medical Care* 29:283–286.

Perrow, Charles. 1986. *Complex Organizations: A Critical Essay.* New York: McGraw-Hill, Inc.

———. 1967. "A Framework for Comparative Organizational Analysis." *American Sociological Review* 32:194–208.

Pfeffer, Jeffrey and Gerald Salanzick. 1978. *The External Control of Organizations.* New York: Harper and Row.

Pfeffer, Jeffrey and Gerald Salanzick. 1977. "Organizational Context and the Characteristics and Tenure of Hospital Administrators." *Academy of Management Journal* 20:74–88.

Phelps, Charles E. 1990. *Health Economics.* New York: Harper Collins Publishers.

Randolph, L., Seidman, B., and T. Pasko. 1996. *Physician Characteristics and Distribution in the U.S. (1995–1996 Edition).* American Medical Association.

Rushing, William A. 1976. "Profit and Nonprofit Orientations and the Differentiations-Coordination Hypothesis for Organizations: A Study of Small General Hospitals." *American Sociological Review* 41: 676–91.

Sandrick, K. M. 1996. "Inside Track: Rural Medicine-Family Affair." *Hospital & Health Networks* (October 20):52.

Scott, W. Richard. 1987. *Organizations: Rational, Natural and Open Systems.* Englewood Cliffs, NJ: Prentice-Hall.

Selznick, Philip. 1965. *TVA and the Grass Roots.* New York: Harper and Row.

Senate Special Committee on Aging. 1985. *Quality of Care under Medicare's Prospective Payment System, Volume 1.* Government Printing Office, Washington DC.

Shortell, S. M. and A. D. Kaluzny. 1994. "Organization Theory and Health Services Management." in *Health Care Management.* ed. S. M. Shortell, and A. D. Kaluzny, 3–29. Albany, New York: Delmar Publishers.

Shortell, S. M. 1988. "The Evolution of Hospital Systems: Unfulfilled Promises and Self-Fulfilling Prophesies." *Medical Care Review* 45: 177–213.

Shortell, S. M., Morrison, E. M., Hughes, S. L., Friedman, B., Coverdill, J. and L. Berg. 1986. "The Effects of Hospital Ownership on Nontraditional Services." *Health Affairs* (Winter):97–111.

Shulkin, D. J., Hillman, A. L., and W.M. Cooper. 1993. "Reasons for Increasing Administrative Costs in Hospitals." *Annals of Internal Medicine* 119:74–78.

Singal, B. M., Hedges, J. R., Rousseau, E. W., Sanders, A. B., Berstein, E., McNamara, R. M., and T. M. Hogan.1992. "Geriatric Patient Emergency Visits Part 1: Comparison of Visits by Geriatric and Younger Patients." *Annals of Emergency Medicine* 21:802–807.

Sloan, Frank A., and Edmund R. Becker. 1984. "Cross Subsidies and Payment for Hospital Care." *Journal of Health Politics, Policy and Law* 8:660–85.

Sloan, F. A. and E. R. Becker. 1981. "Internal Organization of Hospitals and Hospital Costs." *Inquiry* 18:224–239.

Sloan, Frank A., Feldman, Roger D. and A. Bruce Steinwald. 1983. "Effects of Teaching on Hospital Costs." *Journal of Health Economics* 2:1–28.

Sorrentino, E. A. 1989. "Hospital Mission and Cost Differences." *Hospital Topics* 67:22–25.

Starr, P. 1982. *The Social Transformation of American Medicine*. New York. Basic Books.

Steiner, C. A., Powe, N. R., Andersen, G. F., and A. Das. 1997. "Technology Coverage Decisions by Health Care Plans and Considerations by Medical Directors." *Medical Care* 35:472–489.

Stern, R. S., Weissman, J. S., and A. M. Epstein. 1991. "The Emergency Department as a Pathway to Admission for Poor and High-Cost Patients." *Journal of the American Medical Association* 266:2238–2243.

Stevens, R. 1989. *In Sickness and In Wealth: American Hospitals in the Twentieth Century*. New York. Basic Books.

Strange, G. R., Chen, E. H., and A. B. Sanders. 1992. "Use of Emergency Departments by Elderly Patients: Projections From a Multicenter Data Base." *Annals of Emergency Medicine* 21:819–824.

Strasser, S. 1983. "The Effective Application of Contingency Theory in Health Settings: Problems and Recommended Solutions." *Health Care Management Review*. Winter: 15–23.

Thompson, James. 1967. *Organizations in Action*. New York: McGraw-Hill.

Thorpe, K. E. 1988a. "The Use of Regression Analysis to Determine Hospital Payment: The Case of Medicare's Indirect Teaching Adjustment." *Inquiry* 25:219–231.

———. 1988. "Why are Urban Hospital Costs So High? The Relative Importance of Patient Source of Admission, Teaching, Competition, and Case Mix." *Health Services Research* 22:821–836.

Tolbert P. S., and L. G. Zucker. 1983. "Institutional Sources of Change in the Formal Structure of Organizations: The Diffusion of Civil Service Reform, 1880–1935." *Administrative Science Quarterly* 28:22–39.

Tuckman H. P. and C. Y. Chang. 1991. "A Proposal to Redistribute the Cost of Hospital Charity Care." *The Milbank Quarterly* 69: 113–141.

Tyrance, P. H., Himmelstein, D. U., and S. Woolhandler. 1996. "US Emergency Department Costs: No Emergency." *American Journal of Public Health* 86:1527–1531.

Umbdenstock, R. 1987. "The Role of the Board and its Trustees." In *Health Care Administration:Principles and Practices*, ed. L. Wolper and J. Pena 51–57. Rockville, MD: Aspen Publications.

U.S. Department of Health and Human Services, Office of the Inspector General. 1986. Financial Impact of the Prospective Payment System on Medicare Participating Hospitals—1984. Washington, D.C.: U.S. Department of Health and Human Services.

U.S. Department of Labor. 1997. *Report on the American Workforce.*

Vitaliano, D. F. 1987. "On the Estimation of Hospital Cost Functions. " *Journal of Health Economics* 6:305–318.

Vogel, M. J. 1980. "The Invention of the Modern Hospitals: Boston, 1879–1930." Chicago: University of Chicago Press.

Wagner, D. P., Wineland, T. D., and W. A. Knaus. 1983. "The Hidden Costs of Treating Severely Ill Patients: Charges and resource consumption in an intensive care unit." *Health Care Financing Review,* 5:81–86.

Waldholdtz, M. 1982. "To Keep Doors Open, Non-profits Act Like Businesses." *The Wall Street Journal*, (December 12).

Weiner, J. P., Starfield, B. H., Powe, N. R., Stuart, M. E., and D. M. Steinwachs. 1996. "Ambulatory Care Practice Variation within a Medicaid Program." *Health Services Research* 30:751–770.

Williams, R. M. 1996. "The Costs of Visits to Emergency Departments." *TheNew England Journal of Medicine.* 334:642–646.

Woolhandler, S. and D. U. Himmelstein. 1997. "Costs of care and administration at for-profit and other hospitals in the United States." *The New England Journal of Medicine* 336:769–74.

Woolhandler, S., Himmelstein, D. U., and J. P. Lewontin. 1993. "Administrative Costs in U.S. Hospitals." *The New England Journal of Medicine* 329:400–403.

Woolhandler, S.,and D. U. Himmelstein. 1991. "The Deteriorating Administrative Efficiency of the U.S. Health Care System." *The New England Journal of Medicine* 324:1253–8.

Yedidia, M. J. 1994. "Differences in Treatment of Ischemic Heart Disease at a Public and a Voluntary Hospital: Sources and Consequences." *The Milbank Quarterly* 72:299–327.

Zald, Mayer N. and Patricia Denton. 1963. "From Evangelism to General Service: The Transformation of the YMCA." *Administrative Science Quarterly* 8:214–234.

Zwanziger, J., Melnick, G. and K. M. Eyre. 1994. "Hospitals and Antitrust: Defining Markets, Setting Standards." *Journal of Health Politics, Policy and Law* 19:423–447.

Index